RABIES

RABIES

In Animals & Man

Geoffrey P. West

DAVID & CHARLES
Newton Abbot

ISBN 0 7153 5704 2

Set in 11/13pt Plantin
and printed in Great Britain
by W J Holman Limited Dawlish
for David & Charles (Publishers) Limited
South Devon House Newton Abbot Devon

Contents

Illustrations

PLATES

LINE ILLUSTRATIONS

Chapter One

Introduction

Rabies (the Latin word for madness) is an acute, infectious disease caused by a virus and transmitted by the saliva of a rabid animal. When such an animal bites, the infected saliva contaminates the wound, and the virus is enabled to gain entry into the body of a new host.

Rabies may be transmitted violently by tooth and claw—a single rabid wolf has been known to bite twenty-nine people—or stealthily at dead of night, as when a vampire bat feeds on the blood of ranch cattle or, without waking him, takes blood from the toe of a sleeping man.

In recent years proof has been forthcoming that rabies may appear following not only a bite, or through infected saliva contaminating abraded skin or intact mucous membrane (such as lines the eyelids, mouth and nose), but also through the eating of infected food and, in very rare instances, through the inhalation of virus particles present in the air of a confined space.

The virus

'Virus' is an old word with a new meaning. Nowadays everyone uses the term in ordinary conversation, when talking of influenza, the common cold, foot-and-mouth disease, and other ills caused by these smallest of parasites. Differing from bacteria in that they cannot multiply except in living cells, viruses are mostly too small to be seen under the conventional (light) microscope, but can be photographed with the aid of an electron microscope. An example of such photography in this book shows the appearance of the bullet-shaped rabies viruses, each only about 0.00018 millimetre long.

While nowadays 'virus' means an infective agent, in past centuries the word implied simply a poison or venom, and biting animals which spread rabies were often thought of as venomous. In the present century, in Africa, members of the Barolong tribes have described the bite of the yellow mongoose as venomous—'like that of a snake, except that the venom takes longer to act'.

A dreaded illness

Although rabies in man may have a long incubation period, extending for upwards of a year in rare instances, the illness itself is usually brief, lasting only a few days. Nevertheless it is one which has inspired dread, not merely because the onset of symptoms is tantamount to a sentence of death, but on account of the symptoms themselves.

These include a feeling of apprehension; a burning or tingling sensation at the site of the bite; an excess of saliva in the mouth (so that the patient may be constantly spitting); intermittent mental derangement which may be associated with periods of mania when bedclothes may be torn to shreds; pain; and convulsions. The name 'hydrophobia' (meaning fear of water, but used in past centuries as a synonym for the illness) derives from the horror which the mere sight of water can bring to the human patient, who may suffer agonising muscular spasms if he attempts to drink.

Vampire-bat rabies

If the victim could but choose, it would be preferable to be bitten by a rabid vampire-bat than by any other rabid animal, since the illness—though fatal—is then of a less horrifying kind; being characterised by an ascending paralysis, with little or no excitement, and no hydrophobia.

Rabies in the dog

The first symptoms to appear are usually fever and a loss of appetite. The first symptom suggestive of rabies may be a change of temperament. Taciturn dogs tend to become friendly; those of a normally gentle, affectionate disposition tend to become excitable and bad-tempered. The animal may also appear restless and apprehensive. The appetite is capricious. Vomiting may occur. A fear of water is *not* a symptom to expect in the rabid dog.

An alteration of voice, sometimes referred to as the 'rabies howl', may be apparent, while in the 'dumb' form a usually noisy dog will cease to bark.

In the majority of cases of rabies in the dog, the change of temperament is followed by the 'dumb' form or stage, in which there is an increasing degree of partial paralysis but little or no aggressiveness. In a typical case, the paralysis causes the mouth to remain slightly open with tongue protruding, and saliva much in evidence. Loss of power in the hind limbs follows.

The 'furious' form of rabies is an intermediate stage which is seen nowadays in perhaps only 25 per cent of cases. Earlier excitability becomes more marked, and the dog may not only snap at imaginary objects but may bite its owner and, if it runs away—a characteristic of the 'furious' form—may bite any person or animal which stands in its way. Although there may be periods of apparent lucidity and docility, the animal is at other times clearly mad, and dangerous. After a few days the 'furious' form passes into the paralytic or 'dumb' stage.

Rabies on the increase

The incidence of rabies is currently on the increase throughout the world. Historically the disease has waxed and waned in cycles at about a hundred years' intervals, and we happen to be living at a time of one of its periodic advances.

There is great concern today over the existence and spread of rabies among wildlife creatures—foxes, bats, skunks, mongooses, wolves, and many others. Such animals act as a reservoir of infection, which they transmit to farm livestock and to dogs and cats, which in turn may infect man.

In several countries dogs and cats, which can easily be vaccinated against the disease, are no longer the principal hosts and do not constitute an important reservoir of infection. Campaigns to control rabies, either on a national or regional basis, have therefore not merely to include mass vaccination programmes for dogs (800,000 were vaccinated in Spain in 1968) but also difficult and expensive operations aimed at reducing to an acceptable level—from the rabies angle—the population of the principal wildlife species locally involved in the spread of the disease.

On the continent of Europe strenuous efforts are being made to reduce the number of foxes, for it is these animals which have re-introduced rabies into several countries which had been free of it for many decades.

Rabies in antiquity

Already by about the year 2300 BC rabies was not only a

recognised disease in ancient Babylon, but had been written into the laws. It was decreed that if a dog were mad, and the authorities informed the owner accordingly, and if he failed to keep the animal in and it bit someone, a specified fine became payable—so much for a freeman, so much for a slave.

Democritus, the Greek philosopher, described the disease in the fifth century BC. Aristotle, who died in 322 BC, also wrote about rabies.

Celsus, a celebrated physician of the first century AD, was well aware that the saliva of rabid animals was 'venomous' and the means of transmitting the disease. He advised the application of caustics to the wound, cupping, and bathing—especially in the sea—for those who had been bitten. Another, later, physician was a firm advocate of throwing the patient unexpectedly into a pond!

In his *Anatomy of Melancholy*, published in 1624, Robert Burton wrote:

> Hydrophobia is a kind of madness well known in every village, which comes by the biting of a mad dog, saith Aurelianus; touching, or smelling alone sometime, as Slenkius proves, and is incident to many other creatures as well as man.

There is no record of rabies shaping history or leaving a vacant throne; nor can one cite many names of prominent people who died of the disease. If the story is to be believed, one of the most extraordinary incidents concerned the death of the Papal Legate, Cardinal Crescence, at the Council of Trent in 1532. In one of its sudden fits of violence a rabid dog strangled him.

Rabies as an excuse

Bitten people apart, there was often a little wishful thinking. 'He who wishes to kill his dog, accuses him of madness,' was the comment—expressed in French—of Eustace Deschamp in 1400; and Nathan Bailey wrote in 1721: 'When one wishes to drown one's dog, one says that he has hydrophobia.'

The poor excuse of ridding oneself of an unwanted dog was, however, a side-issue, and should not distract from the fear inspired by rabies. This fear must on many occasions have prompted people to ask the question: In view of this terrible disease, is it worthwhile having dogs around?

Dr Thomas Spackman put this very question in a medical book in 1613. 'Now then if so great hurt may proceed from dogges, why doe we make them so familiar companions with us, and use them with so great delight, seeing we may endanger ourselves thereby sooner and sorer than we imagine?' But he came down on the side of keeping dogs.

In the eighteenth century

'Lord Robert Manners told me a strange thing this last October 1778,' wrote Mrs Hester Thrale, a friend of England's most prominent literary man of that period, Dr Samuel Johnson.

> He had his favourite dog hanged at the request of all his family because it had been bitten by a cur suspected of madness. He made the men however bury him in a dunghill that was in the farmyard—this was over night—and the first thing he saw in the morning was his old favourite who came to salute him as usual. The heat of the dunghill had, it seems, restored the creature to life, and Lord Robert then insisted he should take his chance. He did so and died of old age eight years after.

This extract serves to emphasise two important points: the fear ('of all his family') that they might themselves be bitten and develop hydrophobia if their dog had, in fact, suffered at the teeth of a rabid dog; and the difficulty or impossibility of knowing whether or not 'the cur suspected of madness' was rabid.

The fear was justifiable, for once symptoms of this disease have appeared, the most that can be done as a rule—even today—is to ease the patient's mortal illness with the aid of drugs. Ignoring for a moment the intensive care which contributed to perhaps the only authenticated human recovery so far recorded, there is no 'cure' and if, in Mrs Thrale's time, doctors still argued about 'infallible remedies' many people must have entertained doubts as to whether hydrophobia, as they called it, could really be prevented.

Of course, a salivating dog, or one mentally deranged or subject to fits is not necessarily suffering from rabies. This fact was appreciated in Mrs Thrale's time, but it cannot have done much towards comforting the bitten person or his relatives.

However, even if the dog *were* the victim of 'canine madness' there was still a glimmer of hope to be gained from the fact—appreciated by Mr Jesse Foot, surgeon, around 1785—that some people escaped the illness through the dog's saliva being 'wiped away by the teeth passing thro the cloathing or by some other fortunate circumstance.' (Did he realise, one wonders, that a proportion of people bitten by rabid animals do not become ill even if untreated? Perhaps he meant to include that possibility under 'fortunate circumstance'.)

Treatment of bitten persons

One of the earliest treatments consisted of cauterisation of the bite wound.

Later, the use of various herbs was recommended. Medicinal preparations contained also such ingredients as asses' milk, child's urine, and the 'stones' of a hedgehog.

Immersion in water, preferably salt water, was highly

favoured by some physicians. In about the year 1600 one, van Hellmont, became greatly impressed with the effects of this practice in Flanders, and described how an old man was 'cured' of hydrophobia by submersion in salt water. He was held under for four minutes, then taken out and dipped twice more, each time for about a minute. Van Hellmont feared that he was dead, but he 'recovered both his life and his senses'.

On another occasion van Hellmont, from the vantage point of a seaside castle in Flanders saw 'a ship passing by it, and therein an old man, naked, bound with cords, having a weight on his feet; under his armpits he was encompassed by a girdle, wherewith he was bound to the sailyard.... One of the mariners said the old man was a Hydrophobid, and had lately been bitten by a mad dog.'

The old man, a cooper from Ghent, was expected to recover, 'such is the blessing of the sea', as the sailor put it. Van Hellmont followed up the case. The unfortunate old man was nearly drowned by repeated immersions in the sea, and it is a wonder that he survived, but he apparently did.

Richard Mead MD wrote in 1720:

> The ancient physicians, who are followed in this by the moderns, advise, where the place will admit it, to enlarge the wound by incision; to apply a cupping glass; to burn it with a hot iron; to keep a discharge from the ulcer by drawing medicines for many days.

'I cannot but say that I think all this severity needless. The design of it is to draw out the poison, but as it has been proved that this immediately affects the nervous liquor, the mischief must have taken place before the application of this kind can be made.'

Dr Mead advised bleeding, doses of liverwort with black pepper, and cold baths—with submersion at the first sign of symptoms, before high fever. This was better, he maintained, 'than stifling a miserable wretch between two feather beds'.

The following appeared in the *Gentlemen's Magazine* for March 1735:

> Mr. Timberlin, a Gardener, at Chelsea, died by the Bite of a mad Dog this month; also a Lad in Suffolk, though both several Times dipped in the Sea; therefore it may be of Service, on this Account, to mention that there is a Powder of Dr. Mead's, sold by the Apothecaries, which is a Specifick against such Misfortunes, was never known to fail.

Unfortunately this last claim was flatly contradicted in the July issue by the following:

> William Jones, a Farmer, at Milton, near Wooburn, Bedfordshire, being last Easter Day bit in the Nose by a mad Dog, immediately took some of Dr Mead's powder, bathed in salt water and drank large quantities of it.' [Symptoms appeared six weeks later, continued this report.] 'He retained the Use of his intellects, except by intervals, to the last, and was so sensible of his approaching End, that he desired, but a few hours before he died, he might be chained down to prevent his biting or hurting any Body.'

Mr Jesse Foot wrote in 1785 or thereabouts: 'Every medicine that was ever given, for the prevention of Hydrophobia from the Bite of a Mad Dog, has failed . . . Excision by a knife of the bitten part is the only sure and certain method of prevention.'

He gave accounts of five cases in which his treatment had been followed. 'None of these patients took medicine or bathed in the sea,' and 'all recovered.' (Mr Foot, as already mentioned, was a surgeon.)

One medical authority, Dr Henry Sully, was insistent upon thorough washing of the wound with water to remove all saliva, and the continued use of warm water, from a height, before excision. Otherwise, he reasoned, the scalpel might take virus to a clean area and only make matters worse. This view was expressed in 1828.

A Dr Vaughan recommended actual cautery of the bite wound, but went rather further than his contemporaries who thought in terms of heated metal or an acid. He advocated dilation of a wound, if small, filling it with gunpowder, and setting light to it. This, he said, 'would secure a free and continued discharge for some time, and possibly the action of the ignited gunpowder upon the poison may have its uses.'

A much earlier medical man, Thomas Spackman, had advised that 'such as are afraid of a hot iron may have a potentiall cauterrie instead', and the ingredients were specified. Emily Brontë was not afraid. 'When a mad dog had bitten her, there had been no fuss; she had walked quietly into the kitchen and cauterised the wound herself.' This and other acts of courage had endeared Emily to her father, Patrick, whose biographers John Locke & W. T. Dixon remarked that she 'had indeed become the son he had longed for'. Branwell had also been bitten by a dog, but the wound had not been cauterised, and his father was apt to think that this might perhaps have accounted for his behaviour.

Several medical men in London during the nineteenth century assured people bitten by dogs that if the latter drank, or attempted to drink, they could not be mad and so no preventive treatment was necessary. It was an unfortunate misconception, since rabid dogs virtually never show fear of water, as do human beings suffering from rabies, and may drink or attempt to do so even in the later stages of the disease.

In the hunting field

Walter Trevelyan, quoted by Dr S. A. Bardsley in 1807, related how his pack had been joined when hunting by a strange dog 'who was soon perceived to be mad, but not before he had bitten many of the hounds'. All those bitten died.

Trevelyan commented: 'No pack when hunting can be said to be entirely safe, as frequently parts of it are out of sight in woods and coverts; some of the hounds are occasionally lost and absent for two or three days, and who can tell what may happen to them? Besides, how much mischief may happen at night from travelling mad dogs which (as you and I believe) will go to the distance of 50 miles from home.'

Dr Bardsley, Physician to the Manchester Infirmary (where in 1794 forty bitten people had been admitted for treatment within a single fortnight), had been impressed by the success of Hugo Meynell in keeping his hounds free from rabies by imposing a period of quarantine on each newcomer before it was allowed to join the pack. In 1794 Bardsley had advocated a similar measure for the control of rabies on a nation-wide basis, and in 1807 he suggested 'universal quarantine for dogs within the kingdom, and total prohibition of the import of these animals'. Had his advice been heeded, the lives of a thousand or two of his countrymen might have been saved, and effective control of the disease achieved very much earlier.

Bardsley considered that if Meynell's assertions were established, there was a strong presumption that the disease was always produced by the bite of an infected animal. He publicised this idea in 1794 when many people—if not most—were under the impression that in the dog the disease could arise spontaneously and *then* be passed on to another animal by means of a bite.

Experimental transmission of rabies from one dog to another had been demonstrated (or re-demonstrated) before 1810, yet a well known hunting man, writing in 1852, declared: 'How rabies arises it is for me impossible to determine, but that it may be caused by want of water, improper food, and long confinement there is, I believe, little doubt.'

The belief in the spontaneous origin of rabies in the dog

persisted well into the 1870s, and possibly accounted for at least some of the opposition to the muzzling orders introduced in Britain during the last decade or two of the nineteenth century.

Rabies continued to cause heavy losses among foxhounds. The *Sporting Gazette* for July 1 1871 carried the following news item:

> Very alarming intelligence has reached us of the outbreak of hydrophobia in several hunting kennels. The Quorn have lost all their entry, and many of the Albrighton have died; whilst, still more serious, fears are entertained for the fate of the huntsman and one of his assistants in the latter pack, both of whom were bitten.

In this year, too, rabies was affecting to some extent the livelihood of farmers. There were reports of cattle dying in Cheshire, and of sheep becoming rabid in the West Hartlepool area. Farmers in many counties experienced rabies in their stock, but in terms of money their losses from this disease were probably very small in relation to those from cattle plague and foot-and-mouth disease.

In the streets

William Youatt, a prominent veterinary surgeon, writing in 1845, commented: 'The early symptoms of rabies in the dog are occasionally very obscure. In the greater number of cases there are sullenness, fidgetiness, and continual shifting of posture.'

Youatt gave an instance of the consequences of failure to diagnose rabies.

> A Newfoundland dog was sent to my residence, evidently unwell, but the nature of the malady was not suspected. There was evidently something very deceptive in the case, or my assistant was unpardonably careless. The

animal was dismissed with a little physic. On the next day rabies was sufficiently developed. One person only was bitten, but the poor fellow became hydrophobous.

Of Dalmatians Youatt wrote: 'They are certainly beautiful dogs, and it is pleasing to see the thousands of expressions of friendship between them and the horse; but in their continual excursions thro' the streets they are exposed to some danger, and particularly of being bitten by rabid dogs. It is a fearful business when this takes place. The coachman probably did not see the affray; no suspicion has been excited. The horse rubs his muzzle on the dog, and the dog licks the face of the horse, and in a great number of cases the disease is communicated from one to the other. The dog in process of time dies, the horse does not long survive, and frequently, too, the coachman shares their fate. I have known at least 20 horses destroyed in this way.'

In the lawcourts

In 1821 a doctor was ordered to pay eight thousand francs to a poor widow whose husband had died of 'hydrophobia' as a result of a bite from the doctor's dog; the doctor knowing that his dog had been bitten by another dog, and not having kept the animal in confinement.

In England there was a somewhat similar lawsuit. The plaintiff was a labourer earning fourteen shillings per week; the defendant a neighbouring inn-keeper, whose dog had been bitten some time previously, since when it had been kept tied up. Unfortunately, it was able to rush out at the labourer's child in the street—the rope being too long—and bit him in the face. A surgeon dressed the wound, and sent the boy to the seaside for salt water baths, but a month later the symptoms of rabies appeared, and the boy died.

The father tried to recover the amount of the surgeon's fee

(£1 6s 6d) and of the undertaker's bill (£6 or £7) from the inn-keeper, who at first agreed to pay and then went back on his word.

Lord Kenyon said in court that *he* would have killed the dog, which certainly should have been properly secured. Damages totalling £36 were awarded to the father.

Youatt quoted—unfortunately without giving the date—the case of a child bitten by a rabid dog at York. The parents, when all hope of recovery had passed, and wishing to put an end to their child's agony, smothered the child between two pillows. They were tried for murder and found guilty, but afterwards pardoned. The intention of the prosecution was clearly to deter others from resorting in future to this centuries-old method of euthanasia practised in cases of human rabies.

The first vaccine

A turning point in the history of the disease came in the 1880s with the development by Louis Pasteur, in Paris, of a vaccine with which he was able to immunise dogs. He demonstrated that, after a series of inoculations, they could be effectively protected against even fully virulent virus when this was injected into them.

The first tentative treatment with his vaccine of a boy, badly bitten by a rabid dog and otherwise inevitably doomed to die, is described in Chapter 7.

Nowadays, in India, over one million doses of vaccine may be required in a single year, in an effort to save the lives of people exposed to infection.

In treating such people, present-day vaccines—like Pasteur's—need to be administered as a course of fourteen or more painful inoculations; and occasionally they give rise to serious side-effects and even, in rare instances, to death. However, rabies research is currently in a very active state and it can be said, without exaggeration, that a revolutionary treatment is in the offing.

The virus revealed

Knowledge has been accumulating, too, concerning the appearance and nature of the virus itself. Pasteur, of course, was working with an invisible organism of which he knew neither the size nor the shape; and it was not until the 1960s that any inkling was obtained as to its appearance. A very good idea of this is conveyed by the illustration of a model of the virus on page 33.

In 1936 its approximate size had been estimated by means of filtration experiments, carried out at the National Institute of Medical Research, London, by Dr I. A. Galloway and Dr N. J. Elford.

In 1962 Dr Seiichi Matsumoto, using an electron miscroscope at the Institute for Virus Research, Kyoto University, Japan, found elongated particles in mouse nerve cells infected with the rabies virus; and from Paris the Pasteur Institute reported the presence in cells of bullet-shaped particles. Dr J. D. Almeida and his colleagues described membrane-bound particles with surface projections, and wavy ribbon-like filaments emanating from ruptured particles.

In 1967 Dr Hilary Koprowski, of the Wistar Institute, Philadelphia, gave a description of the virus growing in cultures of hamster kidney cells—bullet-shaped, with spike-like projections on its surface. (A more detailed and technical description of the virus is given in Appendix A.)

It had been accepted for centuries that, once inside the body, the rabies virus permeates the nerves; and in 1965 Dr Richard Johnson, of the John Curtis Medical School, Canberra, reported the results of some experiments in mice, confirming that the virus appears to move centrally via the peripheral nerves, reaching the spinal cord in twenty-four hours.

Recently Dr Lothar Schneider, of the Federal Research Institute for Virus Diseases, Tubingen, Germany, showed that after multiplication in the central nervous system the virus spreads outwards again, not merely along the motor and sensory nerves (which, respectively, actuate muscles under control of the will and convey feeling) but also via the autonomic nerves (those which actuate muscles not under voluntary control but which are concerned, for example, with breathing and the beating of the heart).

A subject of wide appeal

The story of rabies, however, is not one of research alone—far from it; but rather one of interest and importance to every cat- and dog-owner (scientifically minded or not), every farmer, every parent, every traveller, camper and naturalist. All these overlapping categories of people will find their varying interests catered for in succeeding chapters.

Chapter Two

Rabies in Wildlife

About a hundred years ago there was a great increase in the world-wide incidence of rabies, and that situation is now being repeated; with mounting outbreaks of the disease occurring among wildlife in Europe, Asia, Africa, and both North and South America.

As the World Health Organisation's *Chronicle* has stated: 'Rabies is an infection of animal populations; an individual case of the disease in man is only the dramatically visible evidence of this infection.'

Since the rabies virus can produce disease in all, or virtually all, warm-blooded animals, its victims vary from mammals to birds, from cat to camel, from tiny mouse to massive elephant.

Not all species of animal are equally susceptible. For example, only ten per cent of badgers may be infected in an area where eighty per cent of the foxes become rabid. This may be because the virus has become adapted to the fox as a host animal, and is therefore less virulent for the badger; or it could be that badgers as a species have a degree of natural immunity. This is a subject at present under investigation. An animal credited with a high resistance to rabies is the opossum.

However, two opposum cases of rabies were confirmed in the USA in 1969.

Once symptoms of rabies have appeared, the outcome in the wild animal is almost invariably death; but infection without the development of symptoms, and recovery from the illness caused by the virus, are both possible. Indeed, they are characteristic of many cases of rabies in vampire bats. Arctic foxes may carry the virus without showing symptoms, and this would appear to occur also in racoons in North America.

While dogs (including 'wild dogs') are the principal carriers of rabies in Africa, Asia, South America, and the southern part of Europe, other animals constitute the main reservoir of infection in many parts of the world. In several areas the fox has superseded the dog as the most important rabies vector. In other regions jackals, wolves, skunks, mongooses, and vampire bats are involved to a significant extent in the spread of the disease.

Where wildlife rabies is present, vaccination of dogs and cats is desirable even in areas where these animals rarely become rabid; otherwise an avoidable risk of human exposure to infection will continue to exist, since dogs and cats act as transmitters of rabies from wild animals to man, and also to farm livestock.

Wild animals include what are sometimes called the 'maintenance hosts' of the virus, assuring its continued existence, as compared with the 'incidental hosts', such as a man or a vulture in which the infection is likely to be a dead-end one—in that the virus is not transmitted to a further host and so enabled to perpetuate itself.

The current upsurge of rabies abong wildlife ('sylvatic rabies', as it is sometimes called) brings increasing anxiety to public health authorities, especially as it has resulted in the disease reappearing in countries from which it had been successfully eradicated. In Europe, for instance, as Mr A. D.

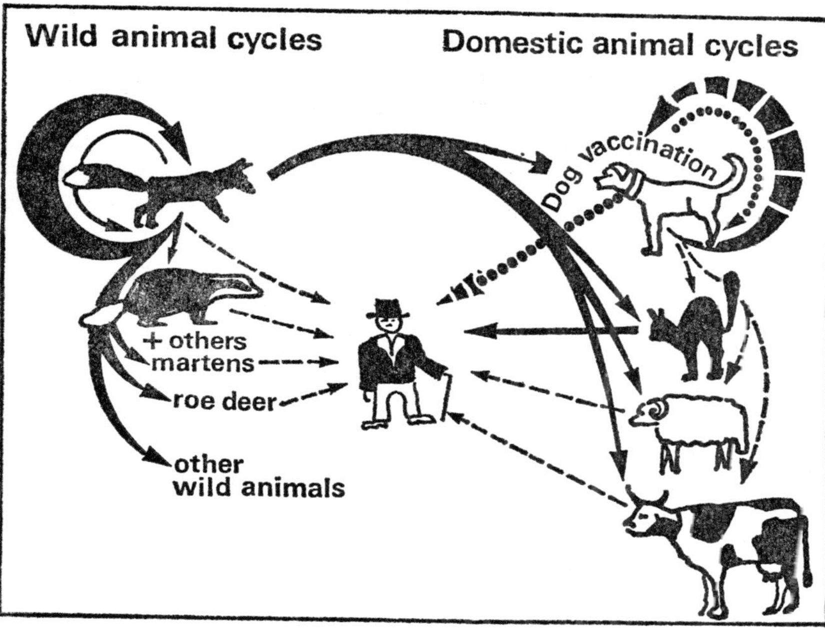

Fig 1 The transmission of rabies, showing the sources of infection in man both from wild and domestic animals in Europe

Irvin has pointed out, it 'reappeared in Belgium after an absence of 36 years, in Luxembourg after 59 years, and in Denmark after 75 years'.

The effect of rabies is often to make nocturnal animals become active by day, and to cause normally timid animals, such as deer, to lose their fear of man and to enter farmyards. In Alberta, Canada, a rabid rabbit went into a farmyard and bit what must have been a very surprised dog! The infection of the brain may also induce rabid animals to travel long distances, thereby taking the disease to wildlife in a district where perhaps it did not exist before.

Wildlife rabies, of course, brought terror and death to

people centuries ago. Throughout Europe wolves savaged many villagers. In France, about the year AD 900, a rabid bear emerged from a nearby forest and reached the quayside at Lyons. Everyone fled at its approach except some boatmen, who attempted to kill it with heavy sticks. The bear, however, bit twenty of its attackers. Six of these became ill with rabies and were smothered (the usual method of euthanasia for rabies patients, and one which persisted centuries later); the other fourteen plunged into the river to escape the bear. Perhaps saliva was washed from their wounds as they swam to the far bank; at any rate, all fourteen survived.

In 1803 there began what George Fleming described as one of the most remarkable outbreaks of fox rabies on record. In several districts at the foot of the Jura Alps people, dogs, pigs, poultry and other animals were bitten. 'Foxes attacked people in the woods, on public highways, even entering villages.' Rabies spread and was maintained by foxes in Austria, Sweden, Switzerland, and in many parts of what is now Germany, and this state of affairs continued until about the middle of the last century when the disease waned.

In Bavaria, two children, a horse, and a steer were bitten by a rabid badger.

At Crema, in Italy, in 1804 a rabid wolf came down from the mountains and bit thirteen people, nine of whom died. In France in 1851 a rabid wolf was reported to have bitten forty-six people and eighty-two head of cattle. The following year, in Turkey, a rabid wolf entered the small town of Adalia, and bit several people in the street, and then—frightened by shouting—entered a garden on the outskirts where, it being the silkworm harvest, many people were sleeping out-of-doors, and bit 128 of them. They could not shoot the wolf, for all firearms had recently been surrendered to the governor. (These figures may of course have been greatly exaggerated, but there is no doubt that wolves will go out of their way to attack human beings when rabid, and that their victims are very often numerous.)

Today rabid wolves still attack people in many countries. Bears have long been in retreat before mankind, and are now (except those in circuses, or 'zoos') usually too remote from civilisation to offer a serious rabies risk except to people such as naturalists, trappers, and members of shooting parties. Nevertheless, in 1967 at least 185 people required treatment after bites from rabid bears.

Campers may be exposed to danger from wildlife rabies. In the USA, not long ago, a rabid skunk entered the tent and then the sleeping bag of an eleven year old boy and severely bit him, with fatal results. Naturalists may become infected through handling a partly paralysed bat.

The danger of wildlife rabies is not invariably confined to the country in which an animal was born and reared. The present craze for exotic pets, the demand for 'zoo' animals, and the even greater requirements of research laboratories, mean that occasionally an animal which is in the incubation stage of rabies is, with its fellows, hunted down or trapped, and despatched to some distant land; there possibly to pass on infection to an unsuspecting purchaser, or to an in-contact domestic pet, or to a laboratory technician. Museum staff may be put at risk by freeze-dried specimens infected with the virus.

In 1965 twenty people had to undergo a course of anti-rabies treatment after varying degrees of exposure to a leopard, sent from Nepal, at Edinburgh Zoo. In London an imported monkey was seen cowering at the back of its cage, biting its fingers and hands. It was destroyed, and rabies was found. Fortunately, this occurred in a medical research laboratory and not in a pet store or someone's home.

Wildlife rabies can be of great economic as well as public health importance. Indeed, in Central and South America where vampire-bat rabies is now regarded as the major cause of death in cattle, it has proved a formidable obstacle to agricultural development and prosperity.

Moreover, countries faced with a serious wildlife rabies problem will, if they tackle it energetically, incur heavy expenditure on control measures. These will include not merely the reduction in numbers of the wild animals principally concerned, but probably also a mass vaccination programme for dogs, and the equipping, staffing and maintenance of laboratories for the production of vaccines and antisera, as well as for diagnostic procedures.

Table 1——
Wild animals commonly involved as rabies carriers:

Canada	FOXES, SKUNKS, Racoons, wolves, bats
USA	SKUNKS, FOXES, RACOONS, Coyotes, bats
Central & S. America	VAMPIRE BATS
Asia	MONGOOSES, JACKALS, Wolves, bandicoots, bats
Africa	FOXES, jackals Polecats, mongooses, genets Ground squirrels, ratels
Europe	FOXES, roe deer Badgers, martens, stoats Weasels, polecats

Table 1 shows the most important wild animals—so far as present knowledge goes—implicated in the rabies problems of different continents. It will be noticed that Australasia is missing from the list. This is because there is no record of rabies in New Zealand; while the last recorded case in Australia was in 1867, at Hobart, Tasmania. Antarctica is also regarded as rabies-free.

'Wild dogs', which are important carriers of rabies in several countries, eg India, are not listed in the table for the reason that international records seldom or never distinguish between dogs and 'wild dogs'. In fact, such a distinction may be difficult to draw, since domestic dogs may revert to the wild state, or become only loosely associated with man; while packs leading a feral existence may scavenge around human habitations.

Domestic cats may similarly revert to the wild state, and become involved in a local outbreak of rabies. In Europe the wild cat (*Felis sylvestris*) and the lynx (*Felis lynx*) are occasionally found to be rabid, but members of the cat family are not generally prominent among wildlife carriers of rabies, at any rate in Europe. In the USA the lynx (known there as the bobcat) has been found rabid in certain parts of the country with increasing frequency.

A large question mark hangs, so to speak, over the rodents. Hares, rabbits, mice, dormice, muskrats, squirrels and voles have all been found infected with rabies virus, but the numbers in Europe had been small until, in 1970, the Czechoslovak authorities claimed to have confirmed the existence of rabies in field rats and mice over a large area of their country. 'Many countries in Europe are concerned about the danger of infection from this source,' the Waterhouse Committee commented.

It should be noted, too, that in the Lebanon rats were in 1969 the second most numerous rabies vector; and a similar position was occupied by rodents in Cameroon, Costa Rica, Guam and Guatemala.

Moreover, bites by rats were given as the reason for vaccine treatment of human beings in a high proportion of cases in the Lebanon, Morocco, and Spain in 1967. In the same year, in Mexico, 500 people required treatment after rat bites.

In West Africa ground squirrels are thought to be important. In India and Thailand bandicoots and other rodents appear to be involved. A report by workers at the Medical Research Laboratory, SEATO Project, Bangkok, stated (1968) that rabies was confirmed in 7·9 per cent of 126 bandicoots (*Bandicoota indicus*), and that evidence 'suggests that the bandicoot rat may be an inapparent carrier of rabies'. Some rabies experts in other parts of the world accept this report with reserve, and would welcome confirmatory work.

In 1970 authorities were stating that there was little or no evidence which assigned to rodents a major role in the spread of rabies although, as Mr A. D. Irvin and others have pointed out, their involvement would explain much concerning outbreaks of the disease. Dr R. K. Sikes stated (1971): 'In the United States we are certain that rodents are not an important reservoir.' Professor Steck comented (1971): 'It does not look as though rabies has an independent cycle in rodents.'

Rodents apart, it should be emphasised that scientific investigation of wildlife rabies is still on a comparatively small scale, still in its relatively early stages. The existence of bat rabies was suspected in scientific circles (as opposed to folklore) only in 1908; and the first isolation of rabies virus from a bat was not made until 1916. In the USA bat rabies was not recognised until 1953.

Nor is rabies always recognised for what it is. In Trinidad, bulbar poliomyelitis was at first thought to be the cause of death in people who died, in fact, from the paralytic type of rabies during the 1925 epidemic there; while deaths in cattle from this vampire bat rabies were at first attributed to botulism.

'Polar Madness', involving the Arctic fox and sledge dogs, and 'Dikovaniya' of Siberia, were identified as rabies as late

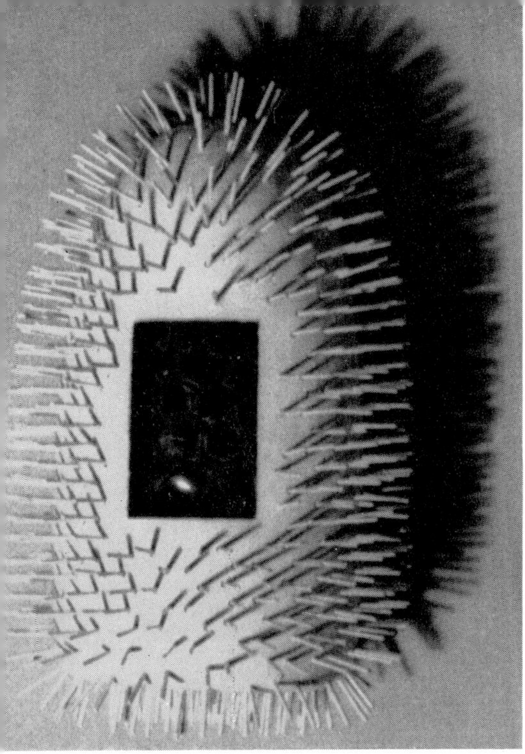

Page 33 (*left*) A model of the rabies virus. The cut away portion is intended to reveal some of the honeycomb-like structure within the virus; (*below*) photomicrograph of the Flury (LEP) strain of rabies virus

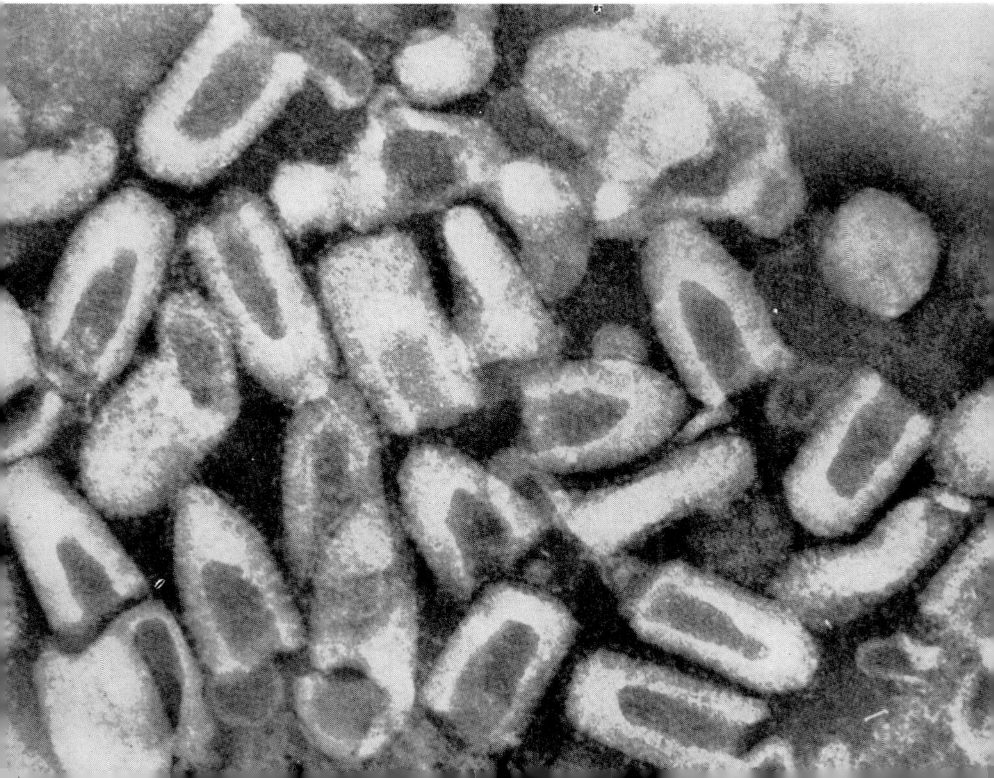

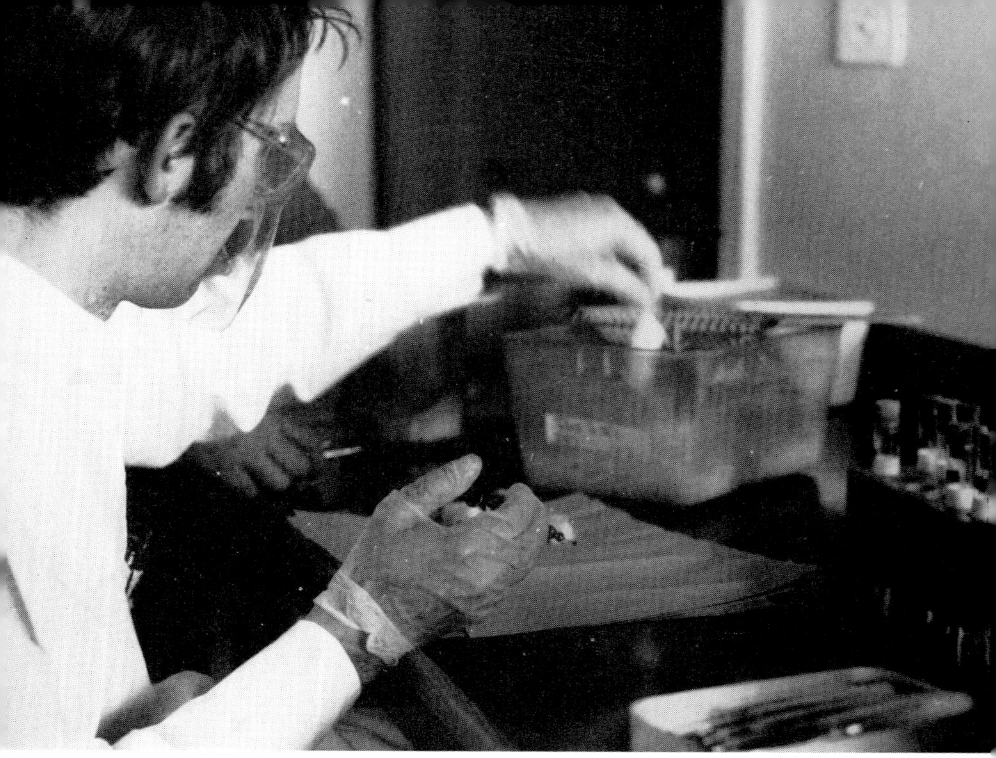

Page 34 (*above*) The diagnosis of fox rabies: a mouse about to be inoculated in the Department of Virology, Veterinary Bacteriological Institute, Bern; (*below*) for the fluorescent-antibody test, a microscope equipped with a dark-field condenser and an ultra-violet light source, in use in India

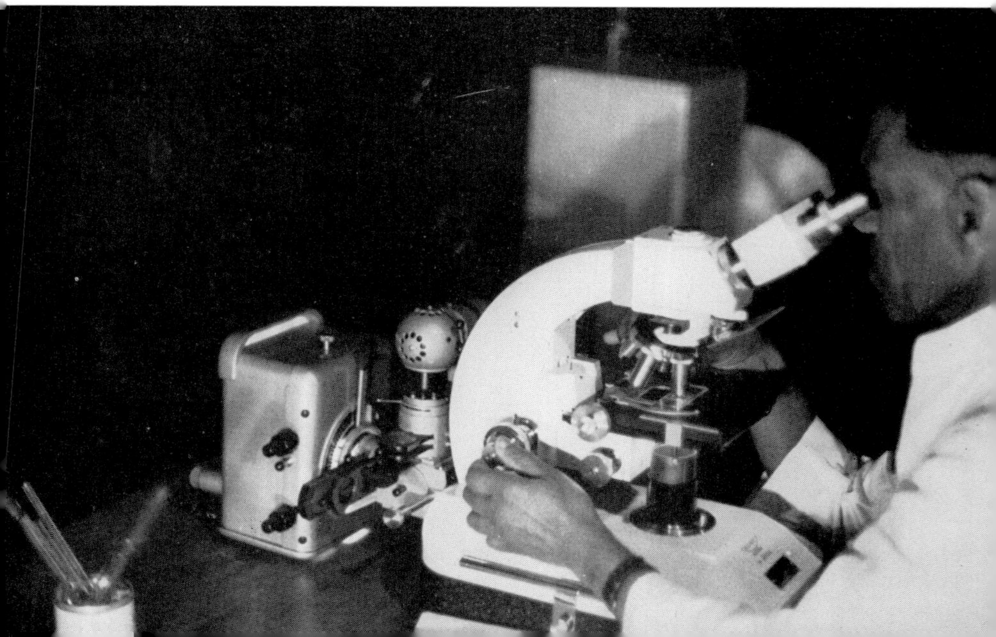

as the 1950s and 1960s. respectively.

Today rabies may still go unrecognised where laboratory facilities—and men trained to use them—are not available for its diagnosis, or where bulbar poliomyelitis seems a more 'likely' diagnosis.

In underdeveloped countries, thousands of villagers may be living far distant from centres where medical services can be obtained. Illness and death may follow a bite from a wild animal without rabies ever being diagnosed or recorded. Even if, after making a long journey to such a centre and being given appropriate treatment, there is no knowing whether a person's death months later in his native village was the result of rabies or not. It follows that accurate statistics are often lacking, and that the number of human deaths from rabies may be greatly underestimated.

EUROPE

On the Continent of Europe the rabies situation has changed greatly since the end of the 1914-18 war when domestic animals—especially dogs and cats—apparently constituted the main reservoir of infection. It was then possible to obtain control of the disease by means of quarantine, vaccination, and the destruction of stray dogs. Control is infinitely more difficult now that history has repeated itself and wild animals have again become the principal source of infection.

Rabies existed among wildlife in the area of the former Polish corridor, where it was found in foxes and badgers in 1939. From there it has spread westwards at a rate estimated by Dr E. Kauker as 40km per year. Rabies spread across the River Elbe in 1950, and reached the Rhine about ten years later. Practically the whole of East Germany, the Federal Republic of Germany, and Poland became affected; together with Belgium, Luxembourg, France, Austria, and part of Switzerland, Czechoslovakia and Hungary.

The animal principally involved is the fox. A 1962 survey showed 767 cases in foxes, as compared with 53 in martens and 52 in badgers. Another report, published in 1968, recorded an incidence of 2·3 per cent in badgers, and 2 per cent in polecats and martens combined, out of 600 confirmed cases of rabies. Out of more than 3,700 animal cases recorded in the Federal Republic of Germany in 1966, over 65 per cent were in foxes; and in 1968 this figure rose to 68 per cent. In Switzerland during 1967-8 the corresponding figure was as high as 84 per cent

Other animals involved are roe deer and, to a lesser extent, weasels and stoats; the lynx and wild cat occasionally. In Yugoslavia wolves become rabid, and these animals are important vectors in much of eastern Europe. There is at least one report of bat rabies from Yugoslavia; as also from Turkey and West Germany.

In the outbreaks of rabies among foxes up to 50 per cent of these animals may die, but this reduction in numbers is not sufficient to do more than halt the progress of the disease temporarily.

Dr E. Kauker has found that rabies in foxes seems to recur in cycles, with high peaks every three years and intermediate peaks in the autumn, when young foxes disperse, and in winter during the mating season. At both these times social contact among foxes is greater and fights more frequent.

Dr R. Novicky has stated (1968) with reference to European foxes: 'It is possible, although it has not yet been proved, that in some foxes inapparent infection develops without any clinical signs. Such foxes can then form a reservoir of rabies virus in nature.' In Switzerland 777 foxes were examined with this possibility in mind, but all proved negative in this respect.

Cases of human rabies in Europe are fortunately rare. Nevertheless it was necessary in 1966, for example, to subject some 26,000 people in Europe (excluding East and West Germany, for which figures were not available) to preventive treatment against the disease. In Switzerland, between 1967 and 1970, eight people were bitten by rabid foxes, five by martens, and two by badgers; but there has been no case of human rabies in Switzerland for over twenty-two years.

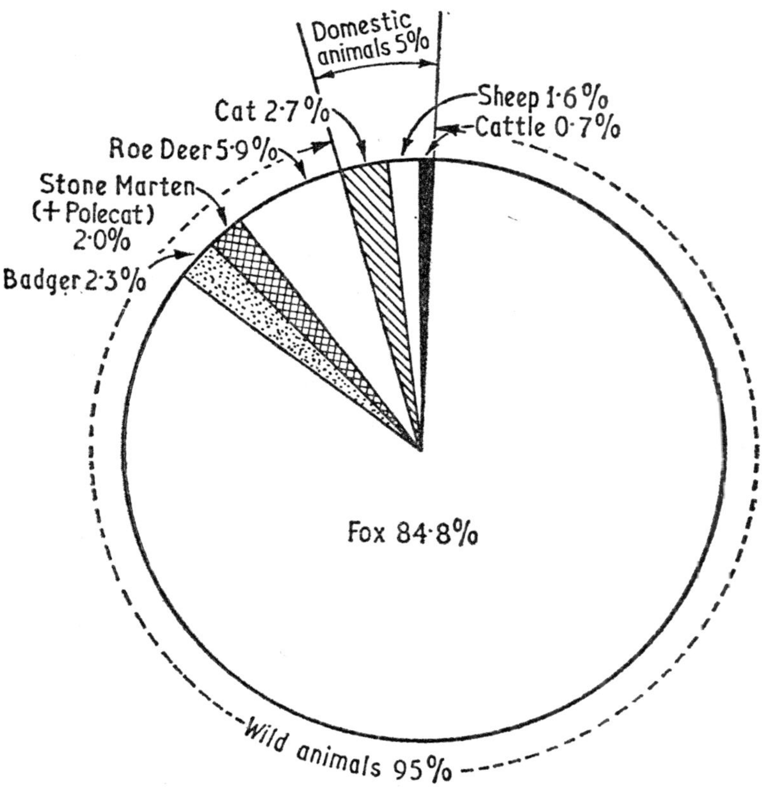

Fig 2 Relative frequency of rabies in animal species

THE UNITED KINGDOM

The serious view taken by the British authorities of the risk of rabies becoming established in wild-life was shown by the energetic but unpopular measures taken at Camberley, Surrey, in 1969. A rabid dog, recently released from quarantine, had been at liberty for a short while on the commons in the vicinity of Camberley. Organised gassing and shooting parties, under the direction of officers of the State Veterinary Service, attempted to exterminate all foxes, squirrels, rabbits, etc., in the area. At the time, this action aroused angry protests from many members of the public, few of whom appreciated the danger, since the disease had not been recorded, *outside quarantine premises*, for forty-seven years.

Strangely enough, there is in modern times no record or evidence of a wildlife reservoir of rabies virus in Britain. Two outbreaks in deer occurred—one near Barnsley in 1856, when nearly 100 head were involved; and another in Richmond Park in 1886, when 257 fallow deer died but did not pass on the infection to red deer nearby. Both outbreaks were apparently caused by rabid dogs. The Barnsley deer were reported to

> foam at the mouth, worry each other like dogs, and tear off each other's hair and flesh and, when placed in a state of confinement, to bite at whatever came within their reach.

At the time of writing, Britain's freedom from rabies continues, but the veterinary authorities realise only too well that susceptible wildlife—including foxes, deer, the polecats of Wales; and such exotic animals as mink and coypu (*Myocastor coypus*) which are now at large in the countryside—could become infected.

Although Britain has the advantage of being an island, there is always the risk of a cat or dog or other animal being smuggled into the country while in the incubation stage of rabies, and avoiding quarantine. Legislation was amended in 1969 to close one loophole—the importation of certain species of exotic animals, eg, monkeys, mongooses, which were previously exempt from quarantine regulations.

There is also the remote possibility of rabies being introduced by a migratory bat. Mr A. D. Irvin refers to a North American species, the hoary bat (*Lasiurus cinereus*) which can migrate over long distances and might reach Britain unaided. 'There is,' he wrote, 'one possible record' of one of these bats in the Orkneys. A specimen of another species (*Vespertilia murinus*) was captured on a North Sea drilling rig, and could possibly have flown from the Continent. However, there is also the possibility that this species and another (*Myotis myotis*) 'which could most easily act as a rabies reservoir on the Continent', are already established in Britain.

CANADA

In the far north of Canada, epidemics of rabies appear to coincide with population explosions among voles and lemmings; giving rise to an increase in small carnivorous animals such as the stoat (*Mustela erminea*). It has been suggested that the latter is perhaps the maintenance host of the rabies virus in the Arctic.

The Arctic fox (*Alopex lagopus*) is an important carrier of rabies in northern Canada (as also in Siberia), and often infects sledge dogs. It is a bluish- or brownish-grey animal with a white winter coat and an absence of the usual 'foxy' odour; and it lives in small communities comprising twenty to thirty adjacent earths (burrows). Below the Arctic Circle the common fox (*Vulpes vulpes*) is the main carrier of rabies.

In Alberta during 1952-4 there was a massive outbreak

among wolves, coyotes (the small 'Prairie Wolf' which often hunts in packs of five to fifteen), and foxes, but control measures on a very large scale virtually eradicated rabies from the province.

Skunks rank next to foxes in importance as rabies carriers; and fourteen cases were confirmed in racoons during 1965-7.

Table 2 shows wildlife animals in which rabies was confirmed in 1966-7.

	Canada as a whole	*Ontario only*
Foxes	519	443
Skunks	224	224
Bats	10	7
Racoons	9	6
Wolves	5	5
Mice	3	–
Rats	1	–
Badgers	1	–

Bat rabies was first confirmed in Canada in 1957, near Vancouver, and by 1969 a total of forty-four cases had been reported. Thirty-two of them were in the big brown bat (*Eptesicus fuscus*) which is an insect-eater and usually a permanent resident. Two others, the hoary bat and the red bat, may migrate in winter which they then spend south of the Canadian frontier.

Dr V. C. R. Walker, in a paper published in 1969, stated that, during the preceding thirteen years, of some 10,000 people receiving anti-rabies treatment in Canada, 20 per cent had been exposed to rabid wild animals. The proportion of animal cases confirmed was 55 per cent in wild animals, 15 per cent among pet animals, and 30 per cent among farm livestock.

Human deaths from rabies have, fortunately, been few in Canada; only four being recorded between 1947-68. Two were in untreated children bitten by skunks, one was in a child bitten by a cat, and the fourth in a farmer who had tended a rabid cow.

During 1966-7 Canada's laboratories found over 1,400 specimens positive for rabies out of the much greater number which they examined.

THE UNITED STATES OF AMERICA

Although in the USA there were only eleven recorded human deaths from rabies during the period 1963-70, some 30,000 people have to undergo preventive treatment every year. While the campaign to reduce the incidence of rabies in dogs has been outstandingly successful, the wildlife rabies problem has grown, as the graph on page 42 shows.

Rabies in skunks and foxes has been a public health hazard in the USA since early in the nineteenth century. Cowboys and buffalo hunters and other rural workers were attacked by skunks—normally harmless and even affable creatures—and in 1870 there were sixteen human deaths following bites from skunks in the Arkansas Valley. The species involved then was, it seems, mainly the smaller spotted skunk (*Spilogale putorius*). Nowadays the striped skunk (*Mephitis mephitis*) is the principal carrier of rabies though, to quote Mr A. D. Irvin, 'this may be more apparent than real, since this species is more closely associated with human habitations than the spotted skunk'.

Skunks now account for the majority of cases of rabies in wildlife, and by 1969 rabid skunks had been found in thirty-two States. References has already been made to a rabid skunk biting a boy camper. A second case, reported in 1970, concerned the death of a four-year-old boy badly bitten by a wild skunk which had been living in his parents' backyard and had

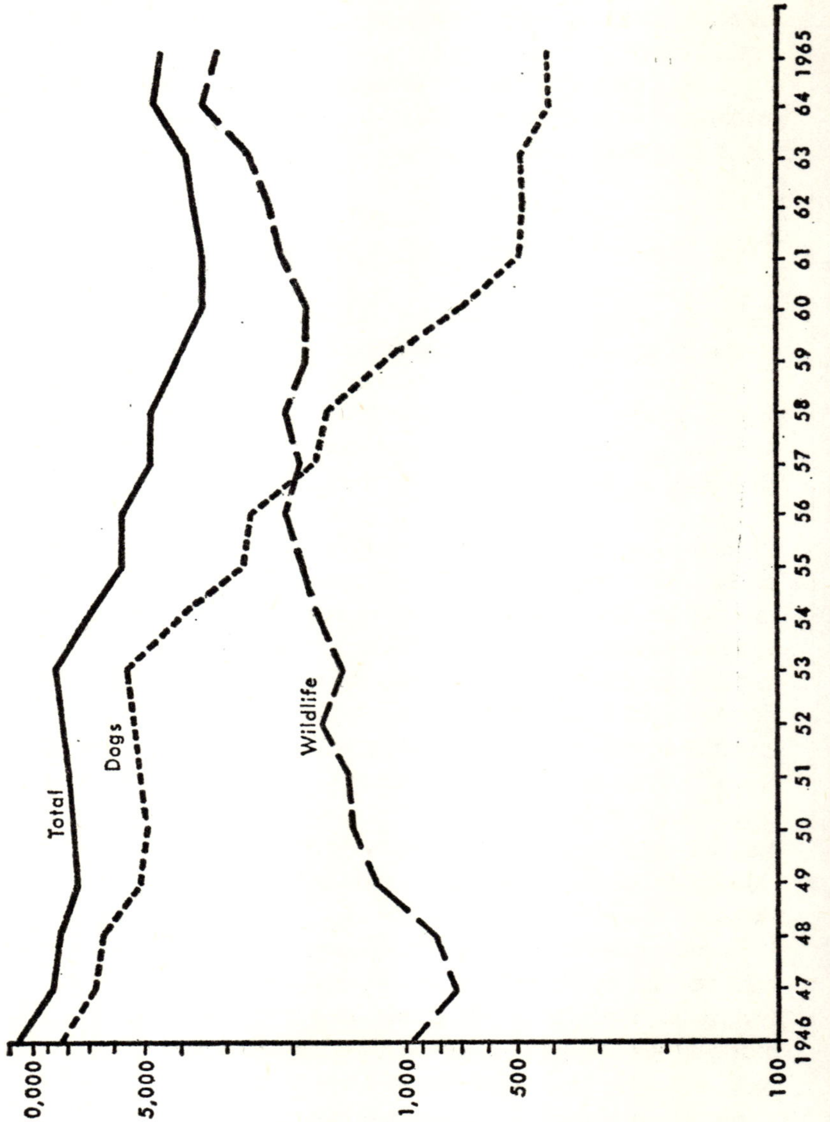

Fig 3 Rabies in the USA 1946-65

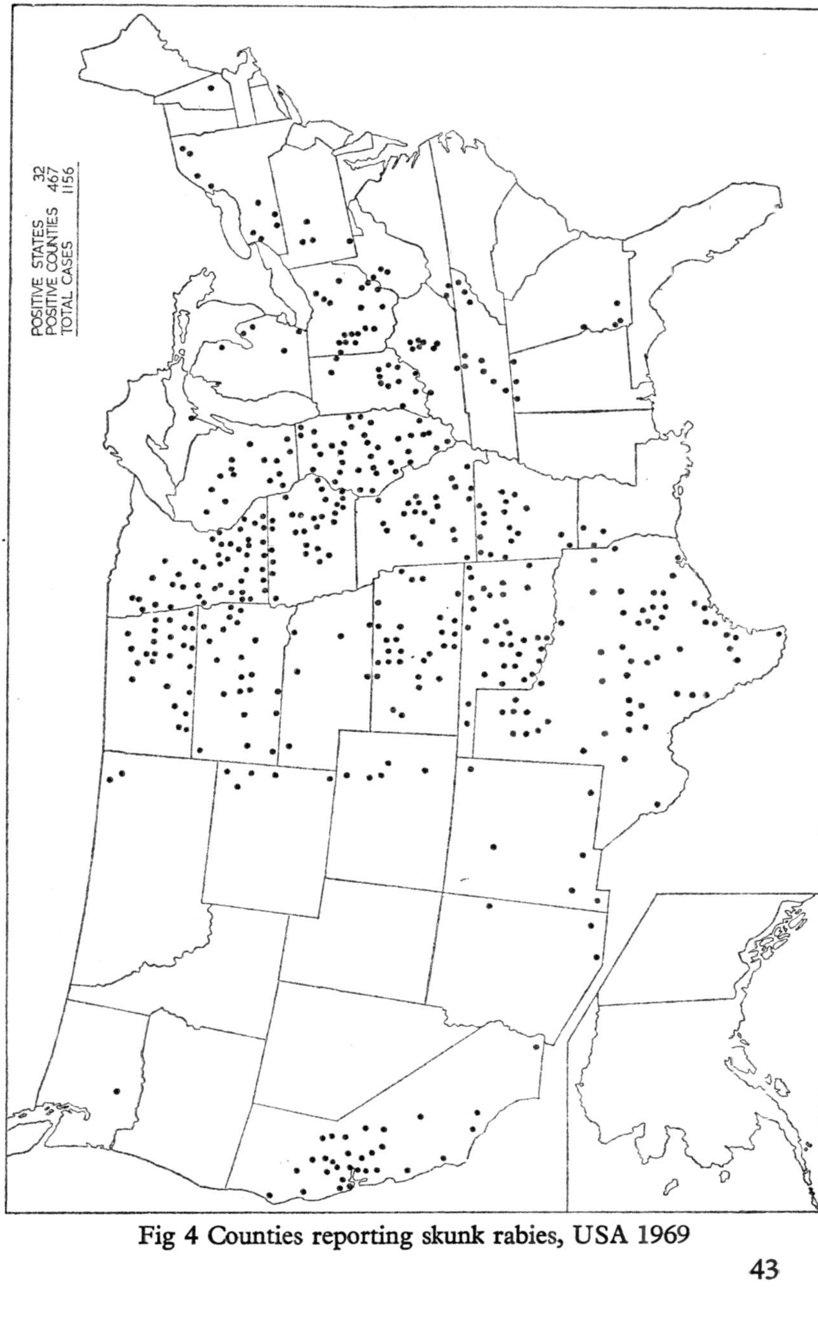

Fig 4 Counties reporting skunk rabies, USA 1969

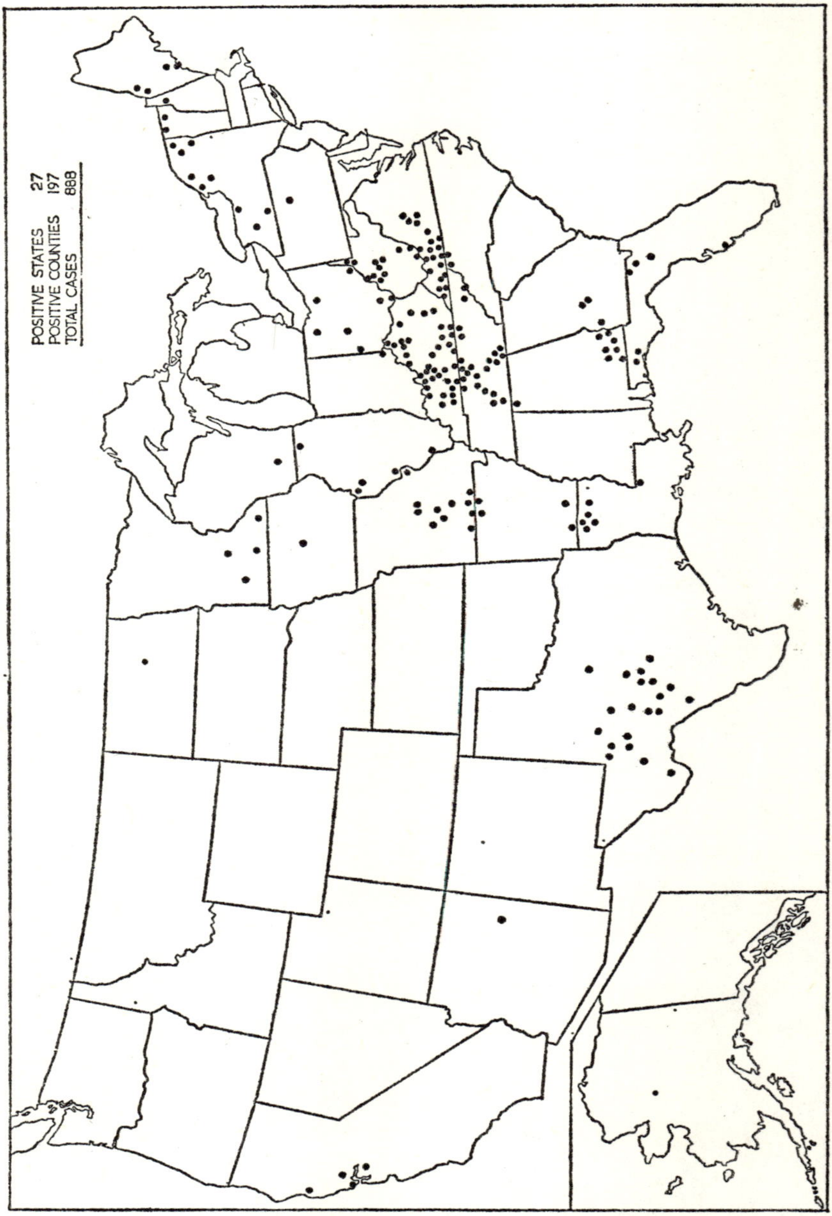

Fig 5 Counties reporting fox rabies, USA 1969

recently had a litter. Skunk and fox rabies caused fourteen human deaths in the USA between 1951-70.

The maps show the distribution of skunk and fox rabies during 1969. The pattern has been changing over the years, with fresh outbreaks bringing the disease into new territory. A 1967 Public Health Report pointed out that during the 20-year period 1946-65 Texas was at first primarily a fox rabies area, but later became primarily a skunk rabies area.

Table 3 shows the principal wildlife creatures in which rabies was confirmed.

	Skunks	Foxes	Bats	Racoons	Coyotes
1958 .	1,005	845	68	50	4
1956 .	1,156	888	321	255	5

Skunk rabies accounted for 33 per cent of wildlife rabies in 1969, and was especially prevalent in California, Minnesota and Texas.

In the same year fox rabies represented 25 per cent of the wildlife total, and occurred in twenty-seven States; notably Virginia, New York, and Kentucky. The common red fox and the grey fox (*Urocyon cinereoargentus*) are the species involved.

In an experiment using virus from a fox's salivary gland, Dr R. K. Sikes found that the incubation period of rabies in the fox varied from 12-109 days; and in the skunk from 14-88 days. The illness in the fox did not exceed three days, while seven out of eighteen skunks showed symptoms for four days; with one exhibiting the 'furious' form for a total of thirteen days.

Rabies in racoons was reported in nine States in 1969; 94 per cent of the cases occurring in Georgia and Florida.

In 1969, in San Diego County, California, a rabid bobcat (lynx) made an unprovoked attack on a 2½-year-old boy, who subsequently died.

Mongooses are important carriers of rabies in Puerto Rico.

Bat rabies was first confirmed in the USA in 1953, after an insect-eating Florida yellow bat (*Dasypterus floridanus*) had bitten a child. Since that time the virus has been isolated from bats in all States except Alaska, Hawaii, and Rhode Island, and from twenty-six of the forty known species of native bat. In 1969 bat rabies represented 9 per cent of the total of wildlife cases.

One authority quotes a Prima Indian as saying, before bat rabies was accepted as a scientific fact in the USA, 'If a bat bites you, you will go crazy and die'.

Unprovoked attacks by bats suffering from the 'furious' form of rabies do sometimes occur, but more often it is when a bat is lying on the ground partly paralysed, able to move but not to fly, that someone—out of curiosity—picks up the creature and is then bitten. Similarly, animals inquisitively nosing a bat in this state are very likely to be bitten. Between 1953-66 five people died in the USA from bat-transmitted rabies.

The rabies virus can survive for long periods in the brown shoulder fat which serves the bat as a source of energy during hibernation; overt disease appearing only after stress has been followed by multiplication of the virus.

Transmission of the virus from bats does not invariably depend upon a bite, nor upon contamination of an existing wound by bat's saliva. Two people died after entering a Texas cave inhabited by vast numbers of bats, and to test the theory of an alternative method of transmission—since neither of these people reported having been bitten—an experiment was made. Coyotes and foxes were kept for one week in the cave, in cages proof both against bats and against arthropod parasites (as possible carriers of the virus). The caged animals became infected. This suggested that the air in the caves was contaminated by virus particles, possibly from bats' urine or

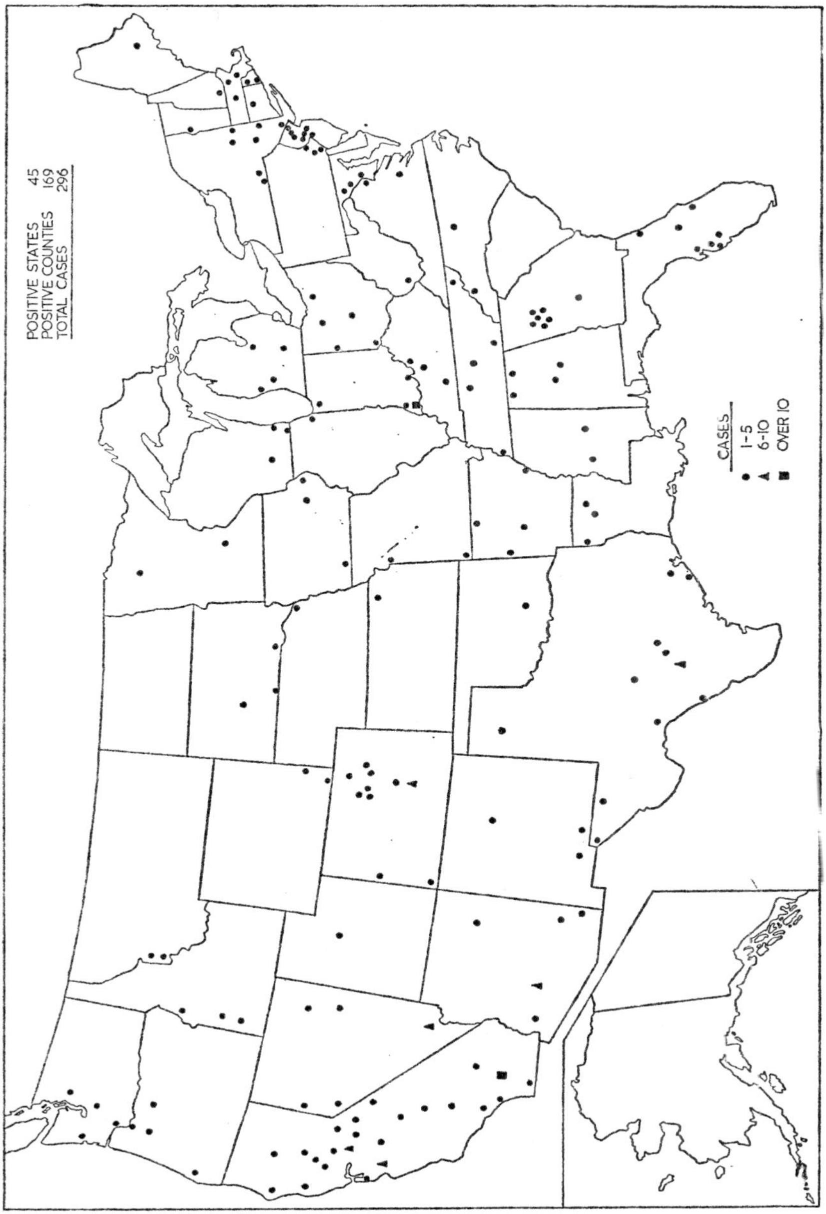

Fig 6 Counties reporting bat rabies, USA 1970

possibly in exhaled air; since the virus can multiply in the kidneys, lungs and trachea, as well as the salivary glands.

The eating of rabid bats is a further possible way by which the disease might be transmitted to foxes, dogs, cats, etc.

The Mexican free-tailed bat (*Tadarida brasiliensis*) is the one most commonly infected with rabies in the USA. It is an insect-eating and migratory bat, and may be an important link in the transmission of rabies from the vampires of Central and South America to other insect-eating bats on the North American continent.

Dr Denny G. Constantine inoculated virus from this species of bat into other bats, dogs, cats, foxes, coyotes, racoons, striped skunks, and opossums. Rabies developed in all these except cats and opossums. 'These results,' he commented, 'are consistent with the suggestion that free-tailed bats may transmit rabies by the bite route among themselves and to certain species of Carnivora.'

The red bat (*Lasiurus borealis*) is also an important carrier of rabies, being found throughout the USA, and especially in the northern States during the summer. It spends the daytime in trees or shrubs. In cold weather it becomes lethargic and vulnerable to predators. It migrates southwards in the autumn.

Other bats which may carry rabies include the leaf-nosed bat, the hoary bat, the silver-haired bat, and the big brown bat. Many carnivorous animals appear, on experimental evidence, to be resistant to rabies virus isolated from the red bat, and from the last named three species.

In 1967 a hairy-legged vampire bat was found among others hanging from the top, inner surface of a disused tunnel in Texas. This was the first report of a vampire bat being found in the USA.

CENTRAL AND SOUTH AMERICA

Dogs remain the principal carriers of rabies in these regions.

However, although the incidence of rabies in Mexico has been on the increase for the past twenty years, mass vaccination of dogs has achieved a reduction in the number of human cases.

In Mexico, deaths (from the paralytic type of rabies) of people and cattle, following the bites of vampire bats, were recorded by the Spanish conquerors in the sixteenth century.

Vampire bats have become numerous in the tropics where, in the words of the 1966 Expert Committee on Rabies, 'large cattle ranches furnish a ready source for the blood meal'; and in Mexico, as in Brazil, Surinam, and the islands of Trinidad and Tobago, vampire bats continue to be important wildlife carriers of rabies.

Vampires live exclusively on blood, a fact which distinguishes them not only from the fruit-eating bats of Africa and Asia, but also from the so-called insectivorous bats. These would perhaps be better termed 'omnivorous', since their diet may include insects, honey, fish, and *sometimes* blood.

Vampire bats make a sorry comparison with the monsters of what is often called horror fiction, for as can be seen from Pates on page 85 they are neither large nor very sinister in appearance; nor do they inspire dread in cattle as do warble flies in temperate climates.

Vampires do not suck blood but lap it from the wound made by their sharp incisor teeth. The blood continues to flow, as the bat's saliva contains an anti-coagulating substance which prevents clotting. From their point of view, this ensures a good meal.

While cattle provide vampires with nearly all their blood requirements, horses and other domestic animals—and occasionally bare-footed people—may be bitten. WHO recorded 160 human deaths from vampire-bat rabies up to the year 1966.

The transmission of rabies by vampire bats is unique in that it occurs during normal feeding routine. In other words, the bat does not bite because it is rabid but because it is hungry.

During the course of feeding, some vampire bats are likely to take blood from cattle already infected with rabies, and having perhaps low levels of virus in their blood. This may happen frequently and could lead to the bat becoming a symptomless carrier. Many vampires themselves die of rabies, it is true, but there is experimental evidence to show that some may recover from the illness, while others never show symptoms yet may excrete the virus over a period of months.

The menace of these bats, which not uncommonly spend the daytime in barns and other farm buildings, has led to the mass vaccination of cattle, which otherwise would suffer heavy losses from fatal, paralytic rabies.

The most commonly implicated species is the vampire (*Desmodus rotundus*). Two other locally important species are the white-winged vampire (*Diaemus youngi*) and the hairy-legged vampire (*Diphylla ecaudata*).

The first isolation of rabies virus from a bat in Brazil came in 1916. The animal was a spear-nosed bat (*Phyllostomus superciliatus*) which had been seen attacking cattle. By 1930 bat-transmitted rabies had been confirmed in Paraguay, Bolivia, and Argentina.

In Cuba, Panama, Puerto Rico, Grenada and the Dominican Republic the grey Indian mongoose (originally imported to kill snakes but now virtually a pest in its own right) is the main reservoir of infection.

Wolves are carriers of rabies in Peru. In that country, and also in Brazil, rabies has been found in monkeys and in rats.

AFRICA

Between 1916 and 1947 more people in South Africa were

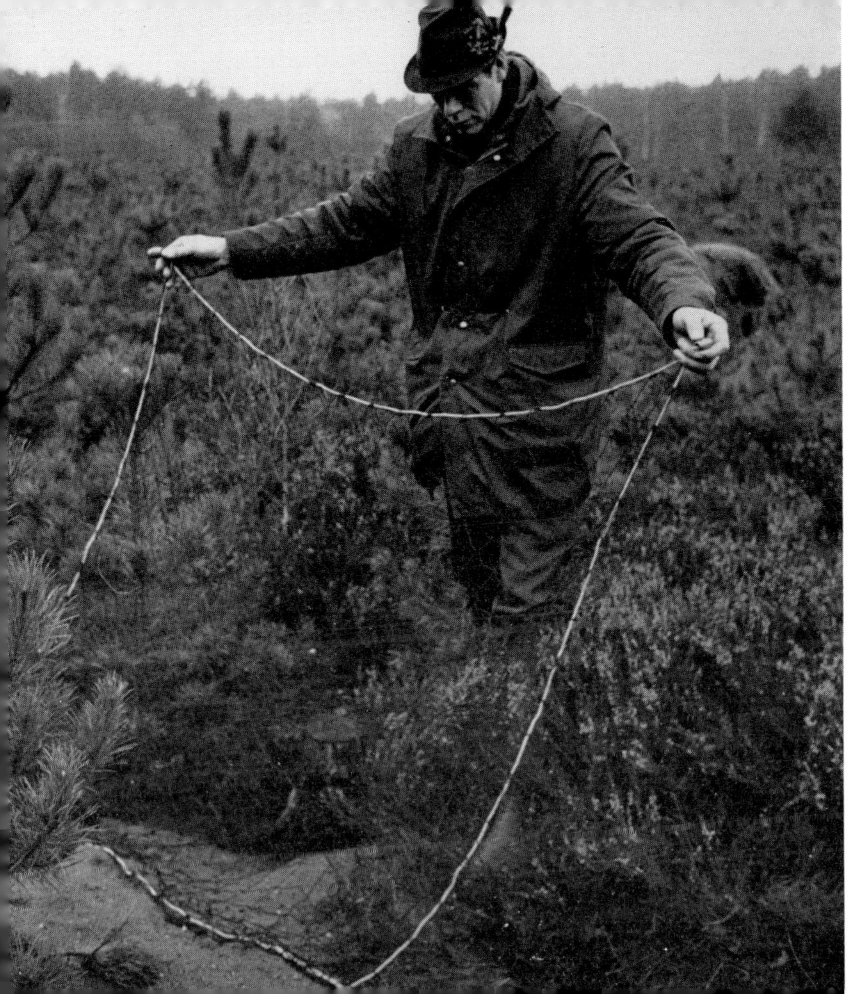

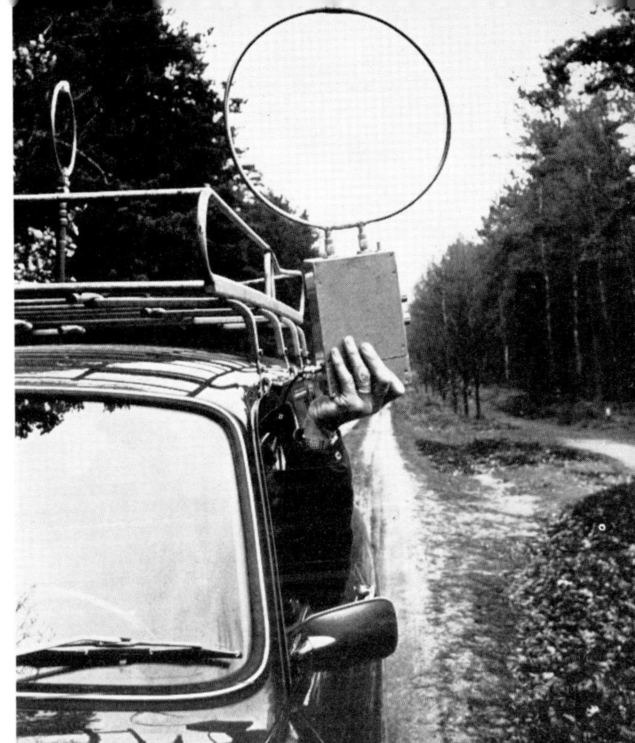

Page 51 (*left*) A game warden in the Netherlands holding a net used to catch foxes for a research programme organised by FAO and WHO to study wildlife rabies; (*above*) radiotelemetry: a device used in a moving car to monitor fox movements in the Netherlands

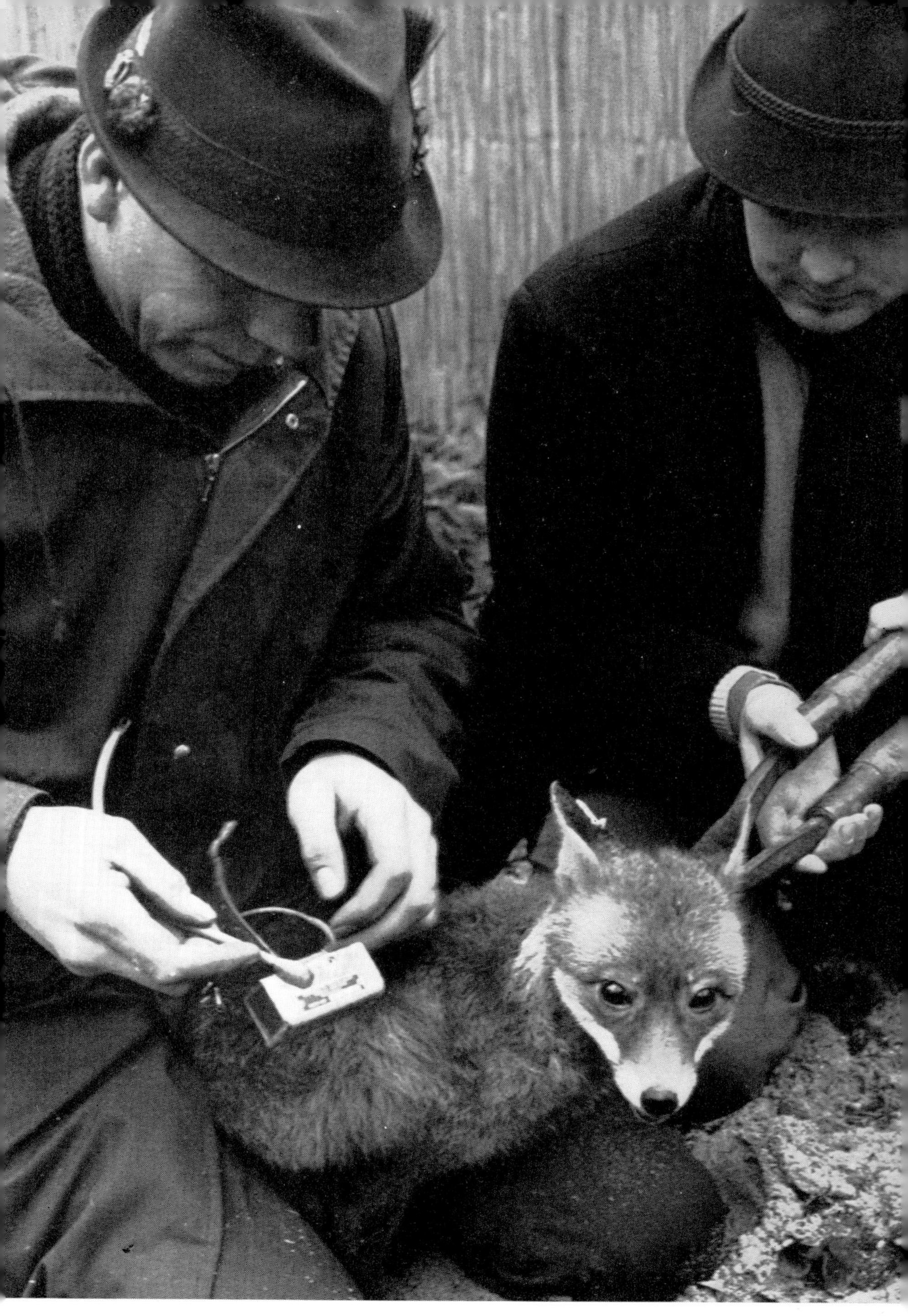

Page 52 After a fox is caught, a radio transmitter is attached to the animal so that its future movements can be monitored by radiotelemetry

bitten by mongooses than by dogs; and of fifty-eight human cases of rabies, twenty-seven followed bites from the yellow mongoose (*Cynictis penicillata*). There is a particular danger to children, who often mistake a rabid mongoose for a tame one, and get bitten.

The yellow mongooses are very numerous in South Africa, and as they live in colonies close to one another, rabies is easily spread. Except in soft sandy soil these creatures are evidently not keen burrowers, and they often share warrens with ground squirrels. The yellow mongoose, also known as the red or bushy-tailed meerkat, may transmit rabies to cattle.

Next in importance to the yellow mongoose is the small, spotted genet (*Genetta genetta*). Other rabies carriers are the Cape grey mongoose, and the common meerkat (*Suricata suricatta*). All these animals belong to the family called Viverridae, and it seems that one strain of rabies virus has become adapted to them; it is present in the Transvaal, Orange Free State, and Western Cape Province.

The second strain of the virus is present in dogs and jackals, and its characteristics were recognised in West Africa in 1947. 'From there', to quote Dr W. O. Neitz, 'it spread through Bechuanaland into Zambia and Rhodesia and Transvaal in 1949. It continued its spread through Mozambique into Natal, Eastern and Western Cape Province.'

One authority has suggested that the yellow mongoose is the carrier rather than the maintenance host, and that another member of the family, the civet, may fulfil this function along with the zorilla or Cape polecat and the white-naped weasel.

Foxes involved include the long-eared Asse Fox or Cape Fox (*Vulpes chania*) and the bat-eared fox, also known as the large-eared Cape Dog (*Otocyon megalotus*). Rabies has also been confirmed in ratels, both in South Africa and in central African territories.

In West Africa, Oulou fato—a disease of dogs—was reported in 1912 to be a type of rabies which runs a mild course, is often followed by recovery, and may exist without any symptoms being shown at all. It is now very widely distributed in Africa, as indicated above. The maintenance host is thought to be not the dog but the ground squirrel (*Xerus erythropus*). This animal has for long had a sinister reputation both in West Africa and the Sudan as a cause of madness and death in people bitten by it.

Table 4 shows the diagnosed wildlife rabies cases in various African territories for 1958.

Algeria	27 rats, 2 mice, 1 rabbit, 4 monkeys
Egypt	3 wolves
Ethiopia	1 monkey
Libya	2 foxes, 2 jackals
Rhodesia	13 jackals, 1 mongoose, 1 badger
South Africa	numerous jackals, 19 meerkats, 4 wild cats

ASIA

Wolves are important carriers of rabies in India and Iran, where thirty and seven cases, respectively, were reported in 1958. In 1969 thirty-six people in Iran had to receive a course of anti-rabies treatment following wolf bites.

Rabid wolves are very fierce in attack and they often bite people about the head, thereby depositing the rabies virus near the brain and increasing the risk of fatal illness. A 1955 report mentioned a single rabid wolf in Iran attacking twenty-nine villagers, four of whom died despite immediate treatment.

Colonel Sir Henry McMahon described in 1935 an outbreak of rabies at Seistan on the Afghanistan-Iran frontier.

The disease was seen first in jackals, next in dogs, and then in wolves. During a single night two mad wolves which had entered Army camel lines bit seventy-eight camels, forty-six of which became rabid.

In India jackals and wild dogs are the principal sources of wildlife rabies. The term 'wild dogs' includes the Southern Dole (*Cyon javanicus*). These are larger than jackals, hunt in packs of six to twenty, and kill wild pigs, deer, and even antelopes. The grey mongoose is probably of less importance in India than bandicoots. These animals are good climbers and have reached, via rainwater pipes, etc, the topmost storey of apartment blocks in Madras, and have been known to fight with dogs after their climb. Ground squirrels are also important vectors of rabies in India.

In Thailand, where there are 400-500 human deaths from rabies annually, bandicoots and fruit-eating bats are among the wildlife hosts of the rabies virus.

Monkeys were found to be rabid during 1969 in Hong Kong, India, Indonesia, and Kuwait. In Indonesia monkeys come next in importance to dogs as carriers of rabies.

In Israel wildlife rabies has involved a mongoose (*Herpestes ichneumon*), jackals, hyena, and foxes; and the badger has been added to the list of potential vectors.

Conclusion

It will be seen from this brief account that wildlife rabies is by no means a straightforward and simple matter, but rather one abounding in complexities and unknown quantities. Perhaps much has yet to be learned about what have been called the 'silent epidemics'—those occurring in species of animals which seldom or never bite man, yet which act as reservoirs of infection and transmit the virus to other species known to be important in the spread of the disease.

The known carriers bite dogs and cats, which bring the infection into people's homes and also re-transmit it back to wildlife. In most parts of the world dogs and cats are important intermediaries in this way, and while mass vaccination of dogs can certainly help, the wildlife problem needs to be tackled in addition. This calls for further study in the realms of natural history and animal ecology—study which will throw more light on the diet, distribution, and fluctuations in population of wild animals living in areas where rabies is present.

Chapter Three

Rabies in Dogs, Cats and other Pets

RABIES IN DOGS

Dogs are the principal carriers of rabies in Africa, Latin America, Asia, and in parts of Europe, eg Greece, Italy, Yugoslavia. In many countries dogs transmit the disease from wild animals, by which they are bitten, to other dogs, to farmyard animals, domestic pets, and to man; and, to a lesser extent, they transmit the infection back to wild animals.

In nearly all countries dogs remain the principal source of infection which necessitates preventive treatment in man, and visitors to a country where rabies is present would be well advised to seek medical aid if the subject of an unprovoked attack by dog or cat.

The insidious nature of rabies is an important aspect of the disease to bear in mind. The illustration of a ferocious-looking dog could mislead the dog-owner into thinking that rabies is always recognisable at a glance. It is not. A capricious appetite, a change of temperament, and a strange look about the eyes may be the only early symptoms observed.

Indeed, occasionally symptoms may not be observed by the

owner at all. An example from North America will show what is meant. A mother, understandably enough, failed to connect in her mind two incidents that occurred on the same day—a slight wound on her baby's lip, and the disappearance from the house of a puppy. The baby later died of rabies, which had not been even remotely suspected. A similar tragedy could occur anywhere in the world where rabies is present—including those countries normally free from the disease but where importation of a rabid animal has reintroduced it.

Symptoms of rabies

After fever and loss of appetite, the illness in the dog is, typically, characterised by a period of melancholy or anxiety, and restlessness. There is often a tendency to hide in dark corners. In some cases bright light causes distress. The animal may vomit. Sometimes muscular tremors may be observed. A change of temperament may be noticed in that noisy, boisterous dogs often became quiet and dull; while those which are normally of a gentle, quiet disposition may become excitable and bad-tempered. The unsuspecting owner is all the less likely to think of rabies if the dog is at times more affectionate. The tone of the bark may alter.

The term 'hydrophobia' as applied to rabies in the dog is misleading, since the rabid dog seldom or never shows *fear* of water (though it may turn away or snap if water is offered) and will often drink copiously and even swim across rivers. Even in the 'dumb' or paralytic stage, when swallowing may become extremely difficult or impossible, fear of water is seldom or never shown. In fact. the dog may rest its muzzle in a water bowl and attempt to scoop water into its mouth.

The symptoms described above may become exaggerated, with increasing excitement, uncertain temper, and a tendency to snap—sometimes at nothing. The dog may run away from home (as the puppy did in the bitten-baby case) before the owner has had a chance to observe any significant change in behaviour. In one language rabies was known as the 'escape disease' because of this tendency to run away.

It should be added, however, that rabid dogs sometimes return home after an absence of a few days. They may by then have lost weight, be covered in mud, and perhaps be blood-stained; and the anxious owner may be very solicitous and approach the animal, with the idea of fondling it or washing it, only to be bitten.

The term 'furious' is applied to this stage of rabies in which there is the tendency to run away (and often to cover distances of up to thirty or forty miles), and to snap at, or bite, human beings, dogs, cats, sheep, etc. Mental derangement is often suggested by the dog's appearance and demeanour; occasionally by its ferocity. There may, however, be lucid intervals in which the animal recognises its owner and is not aggressive.

During this 'furious' stage of the illness, food and water may be taken greedily; or food may be declined, and the dog may swallow instead pieces of wood, coal, metal, carpet, or stones. Vomiting may occur. Occasionally a rabid dog will bite a part of its own body, and there is a nineteenth century record of a dog even biting off its own tail.

It is possible, however, that this was a case of pseudo-rabies (Aujeszky's disease) first recognised in 1902, and giving rise to restlessness, vomiting, salivation, intense itching.

After a very few days, the 'furious' stage of rabies is followed by the paralytic stage.

Paralysis affects especially the lower jaw—which drops, so that the mouth remains partly open, the tongue protruding, and saliva dripping. The muscles of the hindquarters are usually next affected, so that the gait is staggering and the animal falls to the ground. It may regain its feet, but is later unable to do so. Convulsions or 'fits' often precede death.

Early writers on rabies placed much emphasis on the altera-

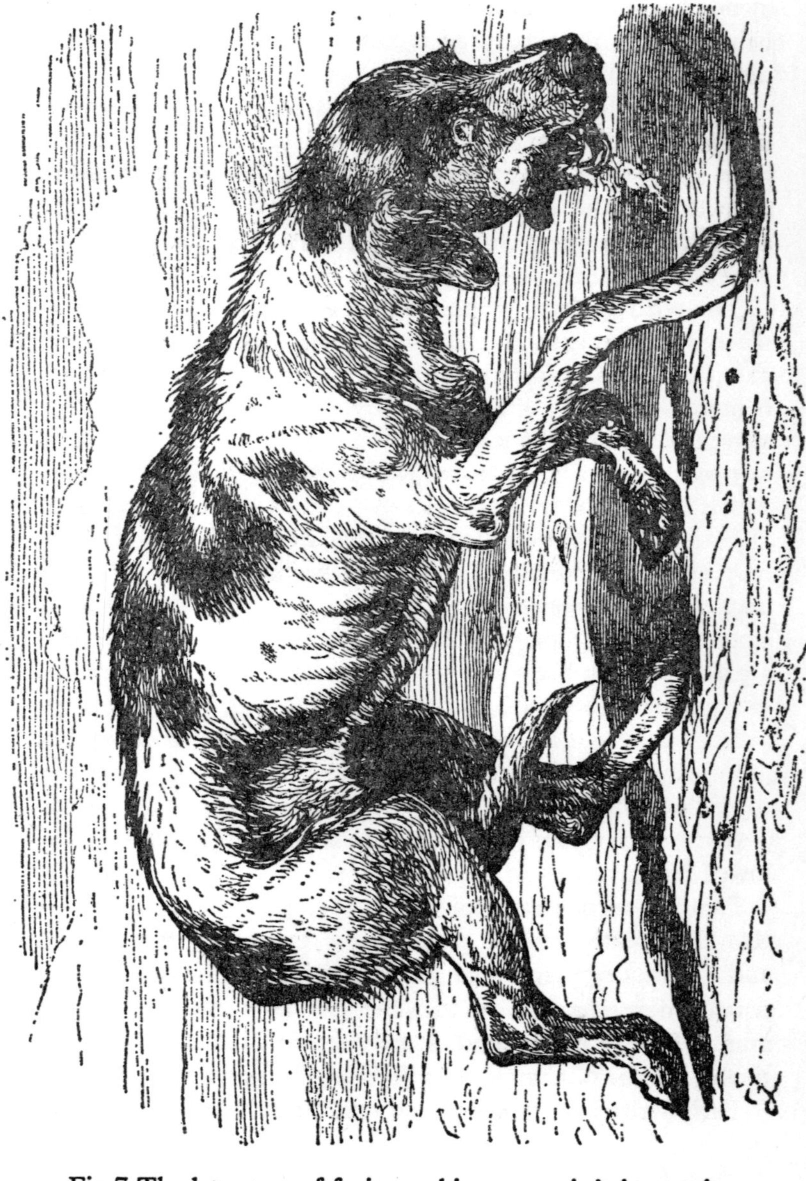

Fig 7 The late stage of furious rabies: an artist's impression

tion of voice during the course of the disease; and this, incidentally, was one of the symptoms shown by the dog Fritz at Camberley. George Fleming related a well authenticated account of how two veterinary students in France were returning to the Alfort Veterinary College one evening when they heard 'the howl of a rabid dog coming from a house'. They felt impelled to knock on the door and warn the occupier of the house; and he, fortunately, taking the warning as seriously as it was meant, kept his large and powerful watchdog on a chain during the night, and next day took it—still docile, affectionate, and obedient—to Alfort, where shortly afterwards it showed unmistakable symptoms of rabies.

In most cases in the dog, the preliminary stage of the disease is followed directly by the third stage. That is to say, the anxiety state or change in temperament is followed by the paralytic stage; and the 'furious' stage is absent. The term 'dumb' rabies has been applied to this form of disease, because paralysis prevents the animal from barking or howling. Excitement, the tendency to run away and to attack, are absent, and the animal remains passive. The tongue hangs out, the lower jaw drops, and there is salivation as already described. The dog's appearance is such as to inspire pity rather than fear.

Sometimes the owner may be moved to fondle the dog and, if it is making sounds suggestive of choking, to put the fingers into its mouth. This can be dangerous, for the saliva is likely to be infective, and transmission of rabies to the owner may occur if the skin of the fingers is abraded.

Finally, it must be added that occasionally a dog is found dead without any symptoms of rabies having been observed. Unless this occurs inside quarantine kennels, rabies will probably not be suspected, and disposal of the body may be fraught with some danger to a person handling it.

Recent statistics suggest that this 'dumb' or paralytic form of rabies occurs in some 75 per cent of cases in dogs; with the

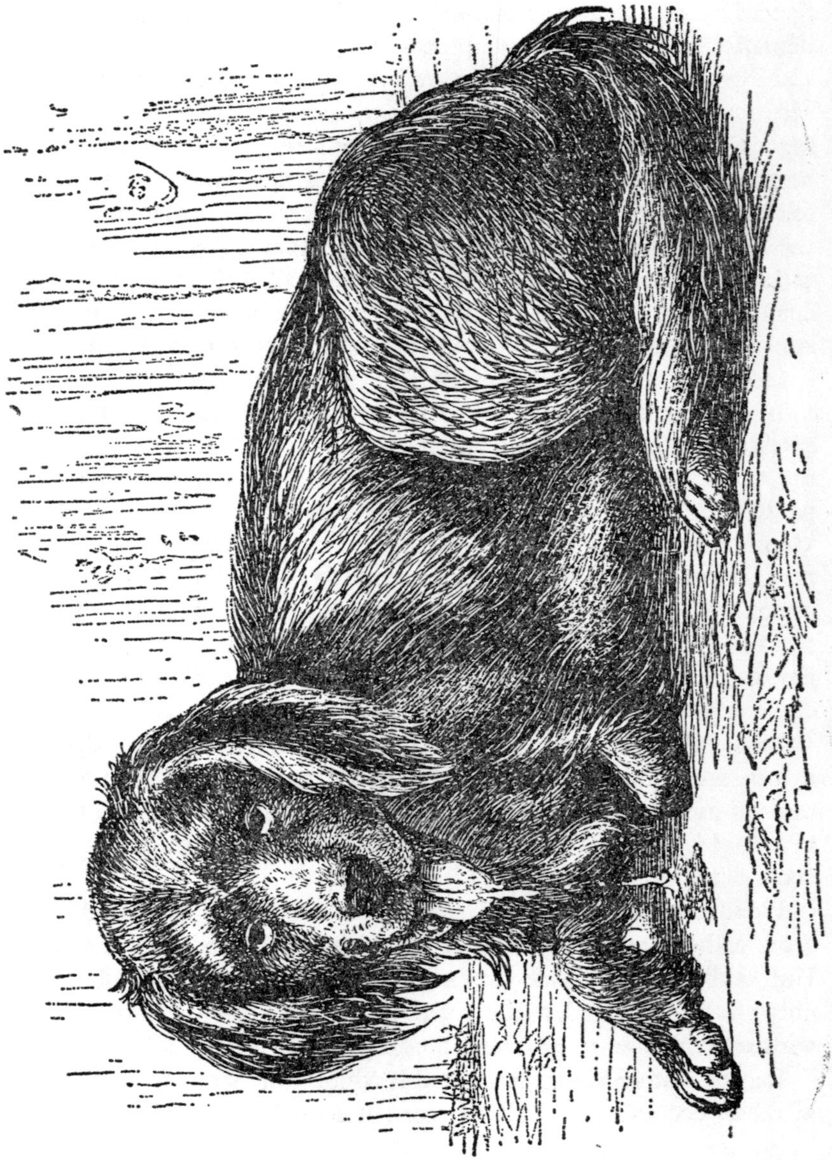

Fig 8 Dumb rabies: drawn from life

'furious' form accounting for only 25 per cent.

Differential diagnosis

A tendency to snap when handled, salivation, a staggering gait, and convulsions are symptoms not only of rabies but also of the encephalitis which is sometimes a complication of canine distemper. Vomiting may occur in the rabid dog; it may also occur—together with convulsions—in canine viral hepatitis. A froth of saliva around the lips may be seen as an accompaniment of 'fits' caused by epilepsy, or by a brain tumour which can also bring about a change of temperament. Convulsions may be a symptom of poisoning, or follow damage to the skull in a dog struck by a car.

Salivation is often profuse when a bone is wedged across the roof of a dog's mouth, or is lodged in the gullet, and the animal may bite its owner if he attempts to investigate. Food and water are refused or, if the obstruction is in the oesophagus or intestine, may be swallowed but returned. This is another condition which may be mistaken for rabies, or *vice versa*.

All this goes to show that a differential diagnosis is called for, and imposes a heavy responsibility upon the veterinary surgeon. He has to bear rabies in mind at all times, even in countries where the disease has not been present for many years, even in a dog which has already undergone six months' quarantine!

In the Camberley case of rabies in 1969, the United Kingdom had been free from rabies (outside quarantine premises) for forty-seven years. It was in these circumstances that an officer of the Royal Army Veterinary Corps was consulted early one morning by another officer concerning his wife's dog, Fritz, which they had brought back from Germany, and which had been out of quarantine for ten days.

This was on a Tuesday. Fritz had been behaving strangely since the previous Saturday morning, when loss of appetite and a refusal of water were noticed. In the afternoon of that Saturday the dog had retired under a bed, coming down to the garden only rarely. On Sunday and Monday it began to make short rushes at its owners, never quite biting them, and then retreating to its position under the bed.

On the Tuesday morning Fritz ran out of the house, cornered a neighbour's cat and, after a bout of hysterical barking, killed it. The dog then fled from the garden, biting the milkman on the shoe, and remained at large for an hour and a half.

By the time that Fritz had been recaptured, the veterinary officer was already telephoning to the Ministry of Agriculture's divisional office his suspicion of rabies based on the symptoms described. When brought to him, the dog 'looked most odd with what I can only describe as an anxious expression on its face'. There was no salivation either then or during the rest of the morning.

Such a prompt warning enabled the authorities to take immediate precautions, which included isolation of the dog, and confirmation of rabies on its death. Other measures included application of the Rabies Order 1938 under which, in the UK, a licence is required for a dog to be taken out of the area, and notified owners must keep their dogs muzzled and on a leash when exercising them. Other legislation was invoked for the impounding of strays. The risk of rabies becoming established among local wildlife was met by an official programme of gassing and shooting of foxes, rabbits, etc, on the commons nearby. On the medical side, two bitten people and about forty-seven others received a course of anti-rabies vaccine inoculations.

A second case of rabies occurred in England in an animal recently released from six months' quarantine. This was at Newmarket in 1970. The terrier-cross bitch, Sessan, had been brought from Pakistan and 'vaccinated three times' against rabies, though precise dates and type of vaccine used were not known.

The history of the illness was as follows. On the first two days the owner noticed that the bitch was not well, though eating and drinking normally. On the third day the animal vomited once. The following day food was refused, although a larger quantity of water than usual was drunk. During the night vomiting occurred three times. On the fifth day she was taken to a veterinary surgeon as 'a vomiting dog which would not eat'.

The bitch was obviously depressed and salivating. No foreign body could be seen or palpated. A closer examination revealed that the lower jaw could not be closed, but when the mouth was fully opened no pain or resentment was shown. Normally this bitch barked a good deal, but had not done so since the third day of the present illness.

Possible causes of the condition were considered to be distemper, gastro-enteritis, a foreign body, poisoning, or rabies. It was decided that the latter possibility required further investigation, and the Ministry of Agriculture's divisional veterinary officer was accordingly informed.

Confined at home, the bitch was beginning to stagger when she tried to walk, and swallowing had become difficult or impossible. Paralysis was complete on the sixth day, when removal to maximum-security kennels was effected. Death followed on the eighth day.

These two case reports, brief as they are, may give the dog-owner a better insight into rabies than a mere recital of all the possible symptoms, which do not all occur together, as a text-book description might suggest. Moreover, as with other diseases, rabies sometimes occurs in forms which are far from typical.

Rabies in Africa

A disease of dogs in West Africa known as 'Oulou fato' was identified as rabies by Bouffard (1912), and this finding was confirmed by means of cross-immunity experiments by Remlinger (1933). The disease is not readily transmitted, as affected dogs show no tendency to bite, as a rule. Oulou fato differs in several respects from the classical form of rabies already described and encountered in Europe, North and South America.

Dr G. Thiery stated in 1959 that in his opinion rabies infection shows different characteristics according to climate and latitude. From observations he made at Dakar on both wild and domestic animals, he declared that the classic concepts of rabies are no longer valid in West Africa.

Rabies in this region is endemic, involves mainly dogs (90 per cent of total cases confirmed), and rarely gives rise to outbreaks spreading rapidly over large areas. The 'furious' form is rare here. The paralytic or 'dumb' form is seen in association with gastritis or gastro-enteritis, giving rise to vomiting; and with the paralysis being of a mild and particular type.

A recurrent form is seen which may affect a dog for three years in succession, at the beginning of the rains. After a period of straying, there is hind-leg weakness. Recovery occurs after the first two attacks, but the third ends with paralysis and death.

A transient form was seen in an experimentally infected dog. Some days after inoculation it became aggressive and showed signs of paralysis. By the tenth day there were signs of recovery, and by the twelfth day the dog was normal. Challenge doses of rabies virus a month and a year later, respectively, were successfully resisted; the animal not becoming rabid. On several occasions symptoms of mild and transient paralysis have been noted in dogs bitten by other dogs (strays).

There are also *healthy carriers* of infection which themselves show no symptoms. (This type of infection has been reported from Russia, India, and Ethiopia.)

In India the director of the Pasteur Institute, Coonoor, received reports of a dog which had seemingly transmitted infection without itself showing symptoms. He was able to trace this animal and brought it back to the institute. Rabies virus was isolated from its saliva, at first fairly frequently but, after several months, only intermittently. This dog showed no signs of illness.

In Ethiopia, Drs Serie and Andral reported, 'abortive' rabies infection may be more common in dogs than fatal rabies. They isolated virus from one dog which was still alive twenty months later. They also demonstrated the presence of neutralising antibodies in the sera of apparently healthy stray dogs.

According to Drs Chalmers and Scott (1969), Oulou fato is probably not confined to West Africa, but involves the whole of central Africa, India, and south-east Asia.

Imported dogs

In Central and South America rabies in dogs is a rarity in areas where bat-transmitted rabies is common in cattle. This may be because the local dogs have acquired immunity or are resistant to bat-transmitted virus. However, a very low incidence of rabies, or its virtual non-existence, in indigenous dogs is no guide as to what may befall the imported dog.

Conversely, the arrival by ship of dogs has in the past often been the means of introducing rabies into local animal populations. The first authentic record of rabies in South Africa, in 1893, associated the outbreak with an imported Airedale. In 1808, according to George Fleming, rabies was taken to La Plata by sporting dogs belonging to English officers. An epidemic of rabies in 1813 in the island of Mauritius was attributed to the dogs on board a ship bound for Bengal.

Long incubation periods

The incubation period of rabies in the dog is commonly between fifteen and sixty days, but periods as short as one week and reputedly as long as a year or more have been recorded.

Long incubation periods are of more than academic interest. They can give the dog-owner an unpleasant surprise after thinking that all danger was past, and they can also breach the defence of even a six-months' period of quarantine.

In a series of twenty-seven cases of rabies inside quarantine kennels between 1924-69 three dogs (two from India and the third from Italy) first showed symptoms of rabies (a) four days before the six-month period was due to expire; (b) after six months and twenty-four days; and (c) six days short of eight months after admission; all three having been retained in quarantine for various reasons.

In the Newmarket case already referred to, it would appear that the incubation period was nine months.

The suspicion that *some* cases of supposedly long incubation periods may have been due to infection from one dog to another within quarantine kennels is discussed in Chapter 6.

It will be readily appreciated that, with animals, it is often impossible to determine with accuracy the incubation period, since there may be no witness of the attack. Moreover, error could creep in if a dog were seen to be attacked by another (presumed but not necessarily rabid), did not itself become rabid as a result of this attack but—unknown to the owner—were subsequently bitten or licked by a second animal and this time did become a victim of the disease. In such a case the owner would naturally assume that the incubation period began with the first attack. Similarly, a person is likely to remember being bitten but to forget a mere lick (especially if the animal was not obviously ill at the time), as Dr H. Koprowski has pointed out in connection with incubation periods of '1-2 years, which need to be critically evaluated', in human beings. Such occurrences may have led to very long incubation periods being incorrectly recorded, but in no way disprove that long periods do, in fact, sometimes occur.

Quarantine and the vaccinated

The reason for refusing to waive quarantine for a vaccinated dog becomes understandable when one considers the Newmarket case. Here was an animal which had been 'vaccinated three times' yet developed the disease. Nor is this example unique. It has also to be remembered that the only 'proof' of vaccination is usually a certificate—which can obviously be forged, issued by an unauthorised person in some far-off country, relate to a different animal, or merely be back-dated.

However, the certificate may be authentic, the vaccine used be one from a reputable company and internationally approved, yet the imported animal may still become rabid. This can occasionally happen because no vaccine, however reliable as a general rule, will protect 100 per cent of the people or animals inoculated with it. There are nearly always a few individuals—perhaps only 1 or 2 per cent—in which the vaccine fails to stimulate antibody production to an extent which will provide a useful degree of immunity. This applies to rabies vaccines as to any other. In Rhodesia, over a ten-year period, rabies was confirmed in 115 vaccinated dogs.

It is, of course, important that highly effective vaccine should not be allowed to deteriorate as a result of too lengthy storage or storage at too high a temperature. It is also important that the interval between doses is the correct one, and that all the doses are, in fact, administered. Two cases of rabies in France were attributed to failure in this respect. In one, the two injections of vaccine were given at an interval of three days instead of the stipulated 15-21 days. In the second case, only one injection instead of the stipulated two which form the 'primo-vaccination' as opposed to the booster dose, was given.

Nearly always, when the disease appears in a previously vaccinated dog, one would expect the reason to be that vaccination had been carried out during the incubation period of the disease—ie, when the dog was already infected; or that there was a failure in antibody production as a result of individual idiosyncracy; or that the level of immunity had declined so that the residual degree of protection was no longer sufficient in the face of a massive dose of virulent virus. Hence the need for booster doses of vaccine.

Dog vaccination succeeds

The foregoing remarks are offered as an explanation of what can occasionally go wrong, and not as an indictment of dog vaccination which is, in fact, one of the most effective means of reducing the incidence of rabies.

British veterinary officers, working in Malaya after the Japanese occupation during the 1939-45 war, achieved spectacular success in controlling explosive outbreaks of rabies by means of the compulsory mass vaccination of dogs and the destruction of strays.

Spectacular success has likewise been achieved in the USA over three decades. In 1946, well over 8,000 cases of rabies in dogs were confirmed by laboratory means. By 1969 dog vaccination, despite a growing incidence of rabies in wildlife, had brought a steady decline in the number of confirmed cases in dogs to 256.

Excellent high-potency vaccines for dogs are available, and

almost all the participants in the Frankfurt-on-Main conference on rabies convened by WHO in 1968 agreed that the vaccination of dogs and cats was a safe and effective procedure which should be undertaken in all rabies epizootic areas. 'Such action protected the human population from the spread of rabies from wildlife through these domestic animals to man, restricting the disease to the wildlife reservoir.'

In countries where rabies is present, dog-owners will do well, in their own and the public interest, to have their dogs vaccinated. The unvaccinated dog runs a twofold risk—being bitten by another (rabid) dog or by a rabid wild animal. In either event, the infection may then be brought into the home.

In some countries, eg Switzerland, Denmark, Germany, vaccination is compulsory, at any rate in some districts, and dog-owners have a responsibility to ascertain what the regulations are, and to comply with them. In the UK all imported dogs are vaccinated on arrival, and this practice obtains at the frontiers of many other countries.

With some vaccines, a single dose will suffice to protect a dog for upwards of one year. Usually, two doses given within certain time limits are required. With inactivated vaccines, booster doses are usually required after one year; with live vaccines, booster doses may be necessary only every other year.

Puppies can be vaccinated when they are a few months old, but will need to be re-vaccinated a year later. Types of vaccine are discussed in Chapter Seven

RABIES IN CATS

In many countries cats are the second source of exposure of human beings to rabies infection; dogs being the principal source. However, in 1969, cat-bite wounds or other contact infection necessitated preventive treatment of people in Belgium, Denmark, Luxembourg and Switzerland to a greater extent than exposure from rabid dogs. In the Netherlands in 1967 one cat (imported from Nigeria) bit five people.

Although usually exempted from compulsory mass vaccination programmes, cats can be effectively vaccinated against rabies without difficulty. Cat-owners would do well to make private arrangements for the protection of their animals and indirectly, therefore, of themselves in countries where rabies occurs.

Much of what has already been said in this chapter concerning dogs applies also to cats. As regards differential diagnosis, it is worth noting that rabies-like symptoms may be produced in the cat by poisoning with benzoic acid. (This substance is used as a food preservative in minced meat sold for dog- and cat-feeding, and poisoning may come about either through faulty mixing or an excessive quantity). Symptoms include extreme aggressiveness; profuse salivation; jumping backwards and striking at the air with the fore paws 'as though catching imaginary mice'; and extreme sensitivity to noise and touch, which may induce fits.

In the rabid cat the change of temperament is not infrequently marked by a show of increased affection.

The 'furious' form of rabies is more common in cats than in dogs; and, as can be imagined, with its sharp claws and teeth which can inflict puncture-type wounds, a rabid cat can be a formidable and dangerous creature. It is very liable to attack both people and dogs.

Nevertheless, in West Germany between 1950-70 twenty-seven cases of human rabies resulted from dog bites; only three from cat bites. In Switzerland, where there have been no cases of rabies in human beings for over twenty years, of fifty people requiring treatment between 1967-70, 68 per cent had been exposed to infection by cats, as compared with only 2 per cent from dogs.

The following table shows the number of people who had to receive treatment in various countries following bites (or other forms of exposure) from dogs and cats. The year was 1967.

Table 5

Country	*Dog bites*	*Cat bites*
Mexico	63,500	3,350
Argentina	23,000	2,089
Brazil	17,490	2,030
India*	31,000	?
Thailand	6,886	95
Hong Kong	1,870	28
Iran	823	57
Lebanon	175	19

(* Figure given from three institutes only)

The following table compares the incidence of confirmed cases of rabies in dogs and cats in various countries in 1958.

Table 6

Country	*Dogs*	*Cats*
India*	50,578	115
Brazil	5,221	498
Tunisia	3,441	182
USA	1,643	353
Algeria	915	0
Turkey	718	12
Peru	274	7
Canada	94	66
Germany, W.	86	91
Ethiopia	68	4
Yugoslavia	56	1
Egypt	43	12

(* Notified by the Kasauli Institute only)

RABIES AND YACHTSMEN

While dogs carried in ships have brought rabies to countries and islands where the disease was previously unknown, it has not surprisingly happened that the incubation period of the disease has sometimes ended before the voyage. Captain Joshua Slocum, famous single-handed circumnavigator, wrote of an incident in his earlier days: 'I have seen the whole crew of a ship scamper up the rigging to avoid a [rabid] dog racing about the decks.'

Sea-going dogs and cats have appealed to those whose favourite reading includes accounts of ocean voyages by yachtsmen. One can recall the Siamese cat and an elderly dog which featured in Brigadier Miles Smeeton's fine books; of the cat Isa Lei which sailed in the schooner *Nordkaperen* during the voyage described by Carl Nielsen, her skipper; of the dog Yo-Yo in *Solace* sailed around the world by Commander Victor Clark RN; of the ominously named Alsatian, Spare Provisions, which was part of a Norwegian crew and shared a shipwreck; and several others.

Rabies was never mentioned, but it would seem prudent that such sea-going animals should be vaccinated. The risk of infection must often be great, especially when runs ashore are permitted in the tropics—or even at ports in temperate climates. To be confined in a small yacht with a cat or dog suffering from the 'furious' form of rabies is a terrifying prospect.

Yachtsmen should, if possible, ascertain in advance the regulations as to quarantine in places where the animal is to be put ashore, and remember that some countries refuse to admit dogs and cats off ships which have sailed from, or called in at, certain ports.

The junk *Golden Lotus*, built in Hong Kong for Brian Clifford, and sailed by him and his crew from there to New

Zealand via Australia, carried a young Chow bitch—a parting gift from the Chinese boat-builder. 'Chow' had endeared herself to the crew, and on one occasion had given warning of an impending disaster, so that it came as a shock when the animal had to be destroyed—since quarantine regulations forbade the landing of any dog from Asia in either Australia or New Zealand.

Indeed, New Zealand would (1971) accept dogs only from Australia and the UK, and then only if the dog had been born there or, if imported from the UK, had been out of quarantine for six months, with no case of rabies in those quarantine kennels during the last three months; and if the dog had been vaccinated against rabies not more than twelve months nor less than one month from date of export.

Exotic and other Pets

In any household, and especially where there are children, rabies in pet animals other than dogs and cats should be thought of as a possibility if (1) the pet is an exotic one; (2) rabies is already present in the country where the family resides.

An example of the imported pet is an ocelot, bought from an animal dealer in Lima, Peru. Although this animal was vaccinated against rabies by a government veterinarian in Peru before being taken to the USA, it died of rabies within a month at San Francisco. Five people, either bitten or scratched by it, had to undergo treatment.

Otter cubs, fostered on bitches, have been exported from India, and in view of the high incidence of rabies there, such pets may represent a risky acquisition.

In 1969, in Yakima, Washington, a four-month-old pet skunk, bought at a pet store, bit two of its owners while being bathed. It died from rabies fifteen days later, and eleven people had to undergo treatment.

As an example of a pet infected by a dog, one may cite the instance of a pet rabbit in Canada which bit two children after becoming rabid. For the most famous case in Canada one has to go back to 1819 when the then governor-general, the Duke of Richmond, was bitten by a captive wild fox and died of rabies.

As an example of a pet infected by a wild animal, there was the free-ranging pet coatimundi in Long Boat Key, an island off the coast of Florida. This animal was bitten and scratched during a fight with what was most likely a rabid racoon—the only other species known to be infected there at the time.

In his paper 'Guidelines for the Control of Rabies' (1970) Dr R. K. Sikes states:

> If people insist on maintaining wild and exotic animals as household pets . . . they should be quarantined for a minimum of ninety days after capture and be vaccinated with a vaccine suitable for that species at least thirty days before being released to an owner.

Elsewhere, the US Department of Health advises that wild animals such as skunks and foxes should be immunised with inactivated-virus vaccine or HEP Canine Kidney Tissue Culture vaccine.

The more exotic the pet, the less likely it is that any controlled trials have been carried out to determine the most suitable type of vaccine for that particular species, or the optimum dose. It would be unreasonable to expect that they had. The vaccination of at least some exotic pets is therefore likely to be a haphazard affair, and owners of such animals should bear this in mind.

Chapter Four

Rabies in Farm Livestock

Cattle are among the species of animal most susceptible to rabies, and in this respect they probably rank next to the fox. In Israel and Argentina they were, in 1969, the species principally affected; and the second species (after foxes) in France, West Germany, and Luxembourg.

In Illinois, USA, during the period 1959-68 farm animals accounted for 13·6 per cent of all the reported cases of rabies. The incidence was greatest in cattle, horses, pigs, sheep and goats—in that order. Skunks were the main source of infection.

The incubation period of rabies in cattle varies from about ten days to several months, with an average length of three weeks. Saliva may contain virus days before symptoms appear.

Symptoms in cattle

The first symptom may be one of depression, but this may pass unnoticed by the cowman and is, in any case, too vague to arouse suspicions of rabies. Loss of appetite and a sudden drop in milk yield in the lactating cow may follow.

The stage of excitement or 'furious' form is characterised

by staring eyes, nervousness, irritability, stamping of the feet, and bellowing. (As rabies affects the voice, the bellow may be of an unusual nature.) Sometimes trembling of the ears may be noticed; or the animal may butt with the head against trees, posts, or other objects. Salivation may be observed, and there may be grinding of the teeth. The tail may sometimes be kept in almost continual motion. There may be sexual excitement, with constipation and straining. The animal may attack people or farmyard animals.

Difficulty in swallowing may lead to dehydration and loss of flesh. After a day or two the cow may become extremely sensitive to noise, touch, or to bright light, and exposure to these may result in convulsions.

In cattle as in dogs the 'furious' form may be absent, and the 'dumb' or paralytic form may follow immediately upon the preliminary stage, so that all that the stockman will observe may be difficulty in swallowing, perhaps salivation, with a loss of muscular power beginning, as a rule, in the hindquarters. Eventually, the animal is unable to stand, passes into a coma, and dies.

Dr P. R. Schnurrenberger and colleagues noted that, out of 97 rabid cattle, 21 had the 'furious' form, 37 the paralytic form, and 39 a form which could not be classified as either. The most commonly reported signs were bellowing (52) and excessive salivation (32). Twenty had paralysis of throat or jaw or appeared to choke. Twenty-one had paralysis of the hindquarters. Eight showed either generalised convulsions or local muscular tremors.

Symptoms in the buffalo, which are estimated to number nearly 120 million and are to be found over large areas of the world from south-east Asia to south-east Europe and parts of north Africa, are similar.

It should be emphasised, however, that all the symptoms mentioned above will certainly not occur in every case, and that rabies is by no means easy to diagnose in the early stages. The following example will illustrate this point.

Differential diagnosis

One January, some years ago, a veterinarian in Iran was called to a large, up-to-date farm some twenty-five miles from the capital. One of the two hundred pedigree dairy cows had been showing signs of nervousness, and muscular spasms or twitchings were in evidence. She was off her food but her temperature was normal. Hypomagnesaemia was diagnosed, and an injection of a magnesium preparation given.

That night it snowed heavily and the farm was cut off, so that the veterinarian was unable to visit his patient again as intended. Unfortunately, she did not progress, but became excitable, attacked some calves and later some men, and broke down part of a calf pen.

On the same day another cow became very noisy and was taken to the bull and served. On the third day, the first cow died, and the second one became violent and was killed.

It was five days from his original visit before the roads were clear again and the veterinarian was able to return to the farm, when two more cows were brought to his attention. The noisiness of one suggested that she was on heat; the other was quiet and friendly, continually coming forward to sniff and lick people. From her nose and mouth hung a little mucus and saliva, but the quantity was slight. Apart from a 'faraway' look in her eyes, and a suggestion of anxiety, she appeared normal.

A second opinion was sought from a consultant to the Veterinary Faculty, University of Teheran, and a colleague on the staff there. To them, although they took a blood sample to be on the safe side, the trouble did not seem to be a metabolic one at all, but rather an encephalitis (inflammation of the brain). A *post-mortem* examination of the slaughtered cow revealed nothing significant, but in view of their suspicion they took away the head for laboratory examination. It proved to be a case of rabies.

Already suspecting this before they left the farm, they had questioned the farm workers, who recalled that a cow had been bitten on the nose some nineteen days earlier by a dog which had visited the farm for a few hours one night and then disappeared. The description of the dog's condition was a further pointer to rabies. (For this account I am indebted to veterinarians W. J. Jordan, MVSc, and M. Hosseinion.)

Given a single rabid dog at large, such an occurrence could be duplicated in any other country. Two points seem of interest. Firstly, rabies was mistaken for hypomagnesaemia during the first visit to the farm, when the only symptoms observed—nervousness and muscular twitching—might well suggest hypomagnesaemia—a common metabolic disease of cattle. Secondly, one wonders if there is perhaps a parallel between the 'quiet, friendly cow' and the extra affection sometimes shown by the rabid cat or dog.

Rabies might possibly be mistaken for another metabolic condition—acetonaemia. In the so-called nervous form of this, loss of appetite is followed by excitement, reckless movements, and an increased response to touch, sounds, or light. A century ago this condition was sometimes known as 'puerperal mania'. As will be seen, rabies and acetonaemia have a few symptoms in common.

Cattle deaths from paralytic rabies in Trinidad, during the series of outbreaks which began in 1925, were at first attributed to botulism, a bacterial infection in which the symptoms may include paralysis of the jaw and tongue, with inability to swallow.

The 'dumb' form of rabies, characterised by paralysis, has led many a farmer to suspect that his cow was 'choking' as a result of a foreign body. Attempts to locate such a foreign body in these circumstances have sometimes proved fatal; for the skin of the fingers may be abraded by the cow's teeth, affording entry of the rabies virus present in the animal's saliva. A farmer died of rabies in Canada in 1959, having infected himself in this way; and there have been other cases since then elsewhere. In 1970, of people treated in Canada, most had been exposed to rabid cattle.

In South Africa farmers have often mistaken rabies for gall-sickness and, in holding the tongue to facilitate dosing the animal, they have exposed abraded hands to infected saliva.

In Argentina, in 1967, thirty-two people had to receive treatment following 'bites or other forms of exposure to infection' from rabid cattle; thirteen after exposure to, or bites from, rabid horses; and nineteen at risk from pigs. WHO figures for the same year in Turkey show that 3,002 bites from farm animals, necessitating treatment of human beings, were notified to the Ankara rabies institute alone; with other cases reported from Istanbul and Izmir.

Cattle themselves become infected with rabies almost invariably as a result of bites about the head or nose. In many countries the chief culprit is the rabid dog; in others the fox. Professor Steck comments that both cattle and sheep often attack dog-like creatures intruding on their pastures, 'and the ill fox may well in some of these instances react in self-defence'. In the USA as already mentioned, the biting animal may be a skunk; while in many outbreaks of rabies in cattle in South Africa there is, to quote Dr P. S. Snyman, 'a history of a mad mongoose'.

Farm livestock which are folded, or penned, or are being reared under intensive conditions, may be more vulnerable to attack by a rabid animal, be it wolf, dog, coyote or cat. One or two American feedlots, where beef cattle in vast numbers are fattened under a zero-grazing system, have experienced heavy losses from a rabid animal gaining entry. Such occurrences are very rare, however, since feedlots are made proof against dogs, etc. Cats are sometimes difficult to keep out.

The table shows the steady decline of rabies in cattle in the USA, where vaccination is carried out only in a few especially valuable animals in high-risk areas.

Table 7

Year	*No of rabid cattle*
1953	1,012
1954	930
1955	835
1956	700
1958	600
1959	700
1960	563
1962	547
1963	459
1969	359
1970	333

In Canada, during the 1952-4 outbreak of rabies in Alberta, 80 head of cattle, 150 pigs, and 25 horses died in the Fort Vermilion and Keg River districts alone. They were mostly infected by rabid foxes, but many were bitten by rabid wolves.

Figures for the whole of Canada in 1967, in respect of farm animals, were: cattle, 417; horses, 15; sheep, 52; pigs, 32.

In Yugoslavia in 1936 a very large number of cattle in the province of Varda were attacked by rabid wolves during a major outbreak of the disease.

In Central and South America, and islands including Trinidad and Tobago, paralytic rabies transmitted by vampire bats had become the major cause of cattle mortality on the ranches there. Before the introduction of a suitable vaccine, some herd-owners in Mexico were losing between 50 and 80 per cent of their cattle from rabies. Mass vaccination has since been resorted to, and over a $3\frac{1}{2}$-year period 2,300,000 head of cattle were immunised with Flury HEP vaccine. More recently ERA cell culture vaccine has been used with great success in several countries of Latin America.

The vampires, which often inhabit barns and other farm buildings by day, bite the cattle at night—on the head, neck or back—puncturing the skin with their sharp teeth, and lapping the blood which constitutes their food. So far as is practicable, livestock buildings are made bat-proof with wire netting; and sometimes bright lights are left on to deter bats.

Horses as well as cattle are preyed upon by vampire bats in Trinidad and Tobago, for example, and it is current practice to vaccinate them annually against rabies.

Symptoms in the horse

The 'furious' form of rabies may occur in the horse, and stable fittings may be bitten—people less often. Paralysis of the throat and of the hindquarters may be seen, with death some three or four days after the onset of symptoms. Rabies may be mistaken for colic (acute abdominal pain) or *vice versa.*

Out of a series of ten cases in Illinois, USA, seven horses had the 'furious' form of rabies, and two the paralytic form. Dr Schnwirenberger mentioned four horses that periodically fell, two that mutilated themselves. Other symptoms: constipation, facial twitch, convulsions, fence biting, incoordination, depression and a dull stare.

In pigs, sheep and goats

Rabid pigs may squeal, become nervous and excitable, but seldom attack people. Twitching of the tail may be noticed, together with spasms of the jaws and of the head. Paralysis follows. Dr L. G. Morehouse and colleagues described an outbreak in which sixteen pigs died at the rate of about two per week over a period of two months. The diagnosis was confirmed by the fluorescent-antibody test and by mouse inoculation. Twitching of the nose, rapid chewing movements, excessive salivation, and convulsions were observed in all these pigs, which were about three months old at the time when losses began to occur.

In sheep and goats, the symptoms may be similar to those seen in cattle; but in many instances little may be observed beyond some form of digestive upset followed by paralysis. A form of 'furious' rabies in sheep in England during the nineteenth century was described as follows: 'The rabid ewes trotted back and forth, biting at hurdles, tearing mouthfuls of wool out of each other, foaming at the mouth.'

Ruminant-to-ruminant infection

Anyone who has had his or her fingers squeezed between a cow's incisor teeth and the dental pad above will know that it can be a moderately painful experience; but with no incisor teeth in her upper jaw the ruminant is not a very efficient biter—so far as transmitting rabies goes. However, not every case of rabies in a ruminant is necessarily a 'dead-end' infection; for ruminant-to-ruminant infection does occur.

Concerning an outbreak of rabies among deer in Richmond Park in 1886, the Appendix to the Report of the Agricultural Department for the following year concluded that the disease was transmitted between the deer by biting:

> It has been found that although the deer attempted to bite one another, they did not really penetrate the skin with their teeth, but only produced sores thereon; at the same time the diseased animals left a certain amount of saliva on the skins of those which were bitten. It was

Page 85 (*right*) Dr Malaga-Alba, a Peruvian veterinarian and bat expert, holding a vampire which has its young one slung from its neck;

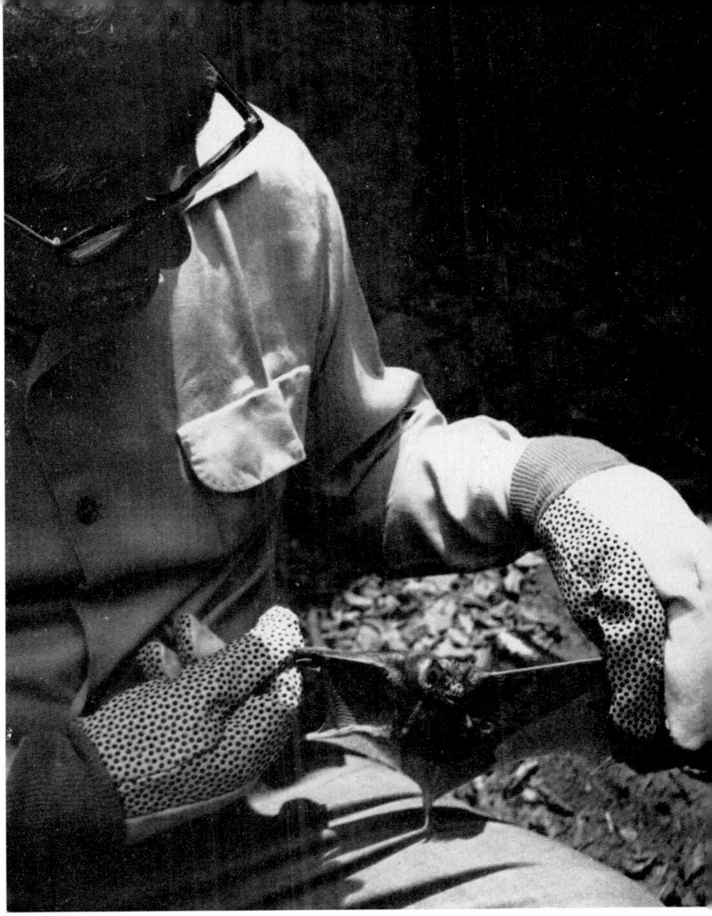

(*below*) a vampire bat such as may transmit rabies in the West Indies, Central and Latin America

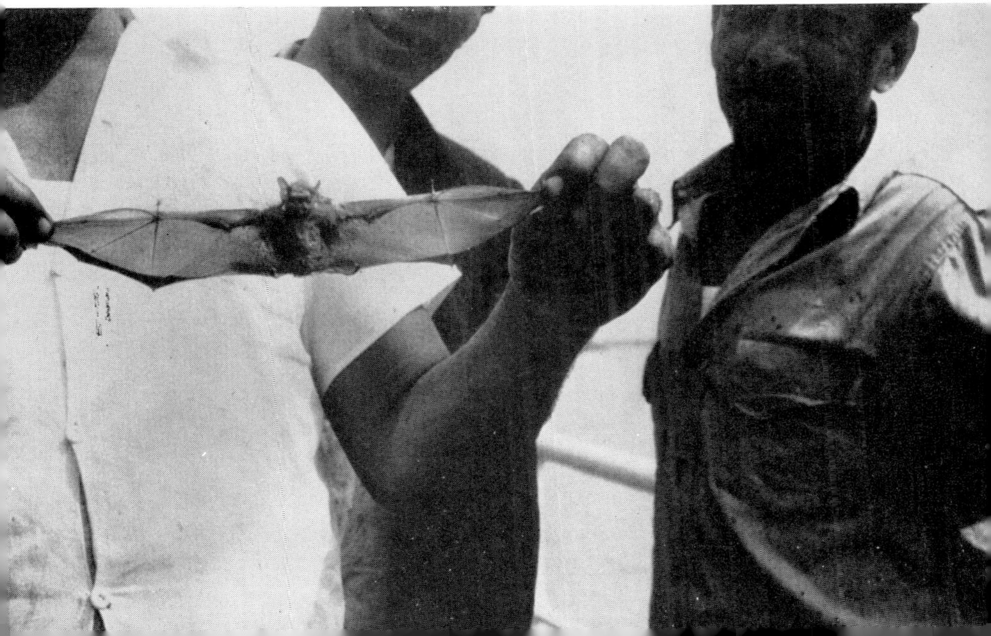

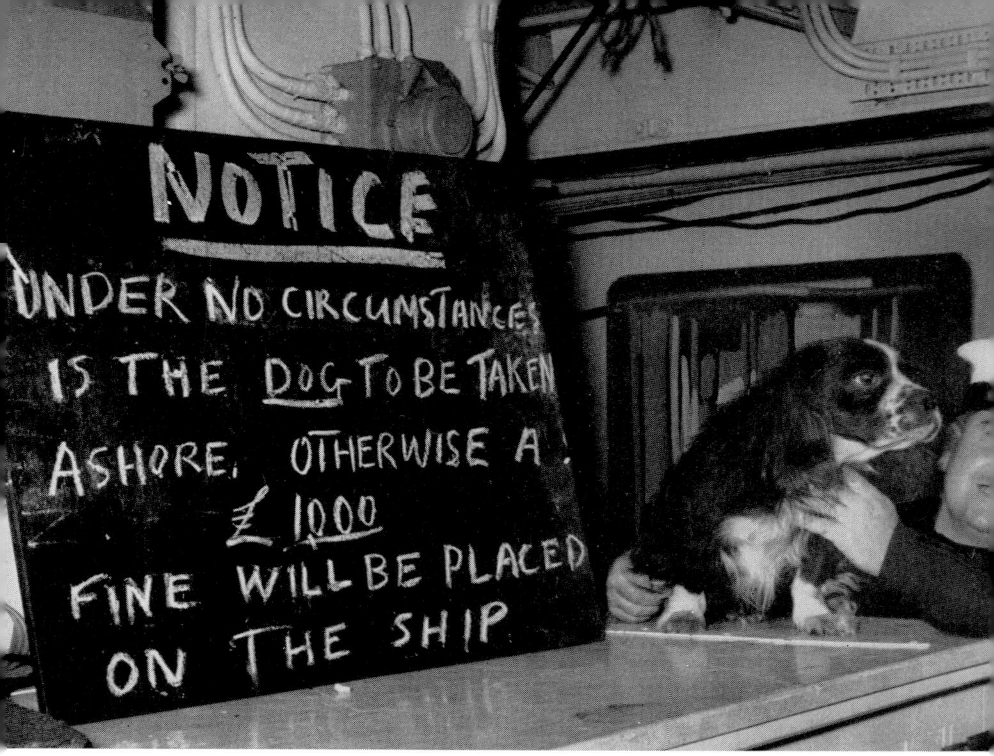
NOTICE
UNDER NO CIRCUMSTANCES
IS THE DOG TO BE TAKEN
ASHORE, OTHERWISE A
£1000
FINE WILL BE PLACED
ON THE SHIP

Page 86 (*above*) A £1,000 fine if the ship's dog goes ashore! A warning notice displayed in the cable ship *Ocean Layer* moored in Greenwich Reach, England; (*below*) dogs brought to a public health office in Guatemala City for free anti-rabies vaccination

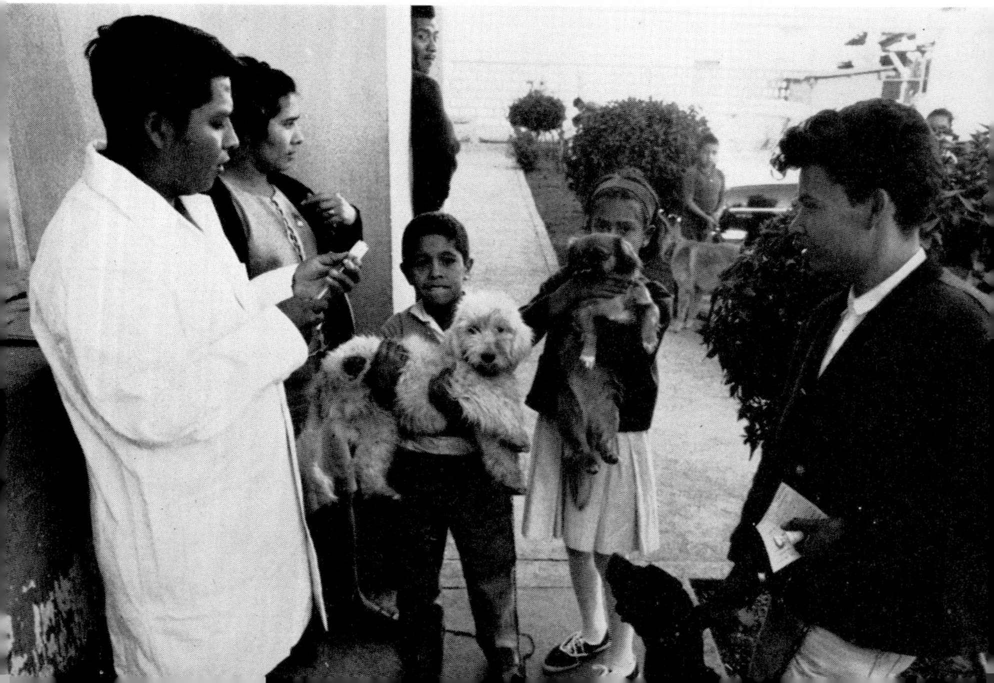

observed on several occasions when a healthy deer had been bitten by a rabid one, that the animal bitten licked the spot, no doubt with the desire to soothe the irritation caused by the pinch or bite, as it is well known that it is a common practice for deer to lick the coats of other deer.

As a means of testing whether the disease could be communicated by a bite, a rabid doe was placed in a shed with a healthy buck, which had been previously entirely isolated from the infected herds. Immediately the rabid doe was placed with the other animal, she flew at it like a dog, and bit it about the ears and neck; the healthy deer was carefully watched, and on the morning of the nineteenth day it showed symptoms of the disease, it became furious, and died in a very short time. This experiment conclusively proves that rabies can be conveyed by the bite of the rabid herbivore to another animal, and was a means of transmitting the infection in this outbreak; the absence of upper incisors in these animals must have rendered this method of inoculation very uncertain in its results, and no doubt accounts for the slow progress of disease among the herd, a circumstance which throughout constituted the most peculiar feature in this outbreak.

A fatal peck

Rabies in birds is only very rarely recorded, but it is worth bearing in mind that domestic poultry are susceptible to infection, and that on occasion a peck from a farmyard cock has led to fatal human rabies. In WHO's world survey of rabies for 1967, there is mention of one person in Argentina requiring treatment after being pecked by a cock.

Rabies and food

In his paper 'Guidelines for the Control of Rabies' Dr R. K.

Sikes recommends that livestock known to have been bitten by rabid animals should be slaughtered immediately. If the owner objects to this course, the animal should be vaccinated and placed in strict confinement for a period of six months. In Denmark, permission may be given for in-contact horses and cattle to be isolated from all other domestic animals and restricted to farm premises for six months; certain conditions being observed with regard to work and while grazing. Cattle and horses subject to these restrictions may be tended only by specially authorised persons instructed in the dangers of rabies and having no uncovered abrasions of the skin. If such an animal dies of rabies, local veterinarians are responsible for ensuring that the premises and possibly contaminated objects are disinfected, straw and manure burnt, and milk safely disposed of.

In Germany, horses and cattle suspected of having been bitten may be kept under official surveillance for six months; pigs, sheep and goats for three months. However, any animal suspected of being infected may be destroyed.

Dr Sikes suggests that an animal can safely be used for human food if it is slaughtered within seven days of being bitten. Persons who slaughter and skin an animal exposed to rabies should wear gloves and take every precaution to avoid contamination from the bitten area. Liberal portions of the tissues surrounding the bite should be discarded. The remaining tissues of the animal he considers safe for human consumption.

Once an animal has shown symptoms of rabies, the carcase should be condemned as unfit for human consumption—likewise the milk.

Farm livestock and quarantine

Throughout the world there is a not inconsiderable trade in

pedigree livestock—horses, cattle, sheep, and pigs—and there is always the risk that an imported animal might be in the incubation period of rabies on arrival. However, rabies is only one of several diseases which most importing countries wish to exclude, and farm livestock will normally be subject to quarantine in the ordinary course of events, so that the rabies risk is usually covered. In 1963 a cow imported from Canada died of rabies in the USA.

Chapter Five

Transmission and Laboratory Diagnosis

TRANSMISSION

The most common method of transmission of rabies virus to man and domestic animals is undoubtedly by the bite of a rabid animal; saliva-contaminated scratches or deep puncture wounds made by its claws providing a secondary route in the case of some species.

Transmission will depend entirely, however, upon the presence in the saliva of the rabies virus at the time the wound or scratch was inflicted. This, of course, implies infection of the animal's salivary glands.

The quantity of virus present in the saliva, the position and severity of the wound(s), and the effect of a person's clothing or of an animal's hair or fur in lessening the amount of saliva contaminating the wound are all factors which (together with the degree of susceptibility or resistance of the host) influence the development or otherwise of the disease.

Infection of the brain and of the salivary glands is often but not always concurrent. If it is, as in many cases of 'furious' rabies, conditions are favourable for transmission; ie the animal has the urge to bite, and the bite can convey the virus.

Professor Tierkel has stated that the rabies virus is found in the salivary glands of between 54 and 90 per cent of animals dead from rabies. Dr R. K. Sikes, in an experiment, found that of 24 rabid foxes, 10 had virus in their saliva; and of 18 skunks, 15 had infected saliva.

Infection of the salivary glands may occur *before* brain involvement resulting in symptoms. In the dog, the virus may be present in its saliva for several days before symptoms of rabies appear. This represents an additional hazard for the owner and other people or animals licked by it; especially if a person's mouth or an animal's muzzle has been licked. In-contact people should be warned as soon as rabies shows itself, and they should seek medical advice. Similarly, veterinary advice should be sought concerning in-contact animals.

Foxes may secrete virus in their saliva for up to 17 days before symptoms appear. For skunks the figure is 18 days, and for insectivorous bats it is 24 days. Further research may show that these are not maximum figures. With vampire bats, shedding of virus in the saliva may occur over a period of several months.

Entry of virus into body

Dr Martin Kaplan has stated (1971) that the virus can penetrate apparently intact mucous membrane, and it is this which lines the mouth, the inside of the lips, the nose and eyelids, as well as the digestive tract. Such penetration explains why a mouth or nose lick may be dangerous, and lends credence to Youatt's account of Dalmatians infecting horses, and Fleming's account of a man's death from rabies after being licked about the mouth by a rabid dog as he lay asleep on the ground.

The danger of infection via the eyes, or conjunctiva (the

mucous membrane lining the eyelids), is tacitly recognised by the recommendation that people carrying out a *post-mortem* examination of a rabid animal should wear goggles or a face-mask.

The unbroken skin is considered to offer an effective barrier to infection by the rabies virus. If a person was licked by an animal subsequently found to be rabid, and the lick involved only intact skin, WHO recommendations are that no treatment in the form of injections of vaccine should be undertaken (but medical advice should be sought).

Existing cuts or abrasions or 'sores' can, however, render a lick dangerous. Henry Sully, MD, in 1807 recorded a case in which a poodle was allowed to lick a woman's face. During the incubation period of rabies in the poodle, she had a pimple —with its top picked off—on her face, and to this fact was attributed her subsequent death from rabies.

Fleming referred to a man who allowed an apparently healthy dog to lick an ulcer on his leg, in the belief (shared to this day in Fiji and elsewhere) that a lick from a dog aided healing. He died from rabies.

Reference has already been made to the danger of putting the fingers or hand into the mouth of a rabid dog, cow, or other animal since, even if the skin was previously unbroken, abrasions may occur through contact with sharp teeth, and if the saliva is infected the virus is likely to gain entry.

By mouth

The eating of meat from the carcases of rabid animals is a possible mode of transmission of rabies to human beings. In 1837 Charles Darwin referred to deaths among some people who had eaten meat from a bull which had died of rabies. Fleming instances a rabid wolf which was killed and eaten by a number of people who all died; and in the present century there have been reports of Africans dying as a result of eating rabid animals.

It is now accepted that, in sufficiently high dosage, the virus can produce the disease after penetration of the digestive tract.

In 1908 two research workers, using a fixed virus, transmitted it to mice and rats by mouth. Fifty years later white rats were shown to be susceptible to oral infection with street rabies virus; and in 1968 Drs Fischman and Ward reported that new-born and adult mice- guinea-pigs, and rabbits all became rabid when the virus was taken by mouth.

It is possible, therefore, that under natural conditions wild animals may become infected through eating rabid prey or carrion. Dr D. G. Constantine and others have drawn attention to the fact that, in the USA, in caves inhabited by bats there sometimes live also foxes, racoons, opossums and wild cats—which will eat fallen bats. Professor Steck has suggested that infection may sometimes occur through eating of infected brains of dead foxes.

Infection could be transmitted through the milk of a rabid animal. The rabies virus has been isolated from the milk and mammary glands of several species of animals. Infection of the suckling bat has been recorded. In practice, it may sometimes be difficult to differentiate between infection via the milk and via the maternal saliva when offspring are licked. Erupting teeth, it has been pointed out, could facilitate entry of the virus through non-intact mucous membrane.

Kidney tissue may harbour the rabies virus, which has been isolated from the urine of several species of animals. Shedding of the virus in fox urine was reported (1966) by Dr E. Kauker, who suggested that the virus could possibly be transmitted to other foxes sniffing the trail of a rabid one. It is interesting to speculate as to whether such a mode of transmission ever occurs in the dog, but Professor Steck states that there is no evidence whatsoever of this; nor has he found the virus in fox urine as detected by mouse inoculation tests.

The possibility of 'indirect transmission' as a means whereby a dog in quarantine kennels may have infected one or two others was raised in the Waterhouse Committee's report, but it was stated that there was no record of such an occurrence involving the dog. 'Indirect transmission' was not defined, but in the context of quarantine premises, where the air would never be stagnant, it presumably could only arise through one dog gaining access to the saliva, urine or faeces of another dog.

Aerosol transmission

Two men who had been into the Frio Cave, Texas, frequented by rabid bats, both died of rabies—one in 1956, and the other in 1959—though neither had reported being bitten. Aerosol transmission is the accepted explanation. The virus may have come from bats' saliva or urine, or conceivably from their breath, since the virus is known to multiply in the cells of the lungs and trachea.

Rabies was confirmed at the rabies experimental station, New Mexico, USA, in animals—coyotes, red and grey foxes, racoons, and opossums—which had been exposed in bat-infested caves in such a way that neither bats nor their parasites could make direct contact.

Dr R. K. Sikes has also reported an experiment in which foxes, exposed to virus dispersed in much the same way as an aerosol, were kept in individual cages in a large room housing unchallenged coyotes, foxes and racoons. Many of these animals died from rabies about six months after the introduction into the room of the foxes exposed to the air-borne virus. Dr Martin Kaplan later commented:

> There is little doubt in the minds of the investigators that air-borne infection had occurred on these premises . . . A

> relatively high concentration of virus may have been present in the circulating air of the room at various periods, perhaps resulting from adherence of virus particles to the fur of the animals.

Mr A. D. Irvin commented that it is possible that aerosol transmission could occur in burrows where a heavy concentration of virus could build up in the stagnant air, 'and in this respect it is perhaps significant that all the important maintenance hosts, except bats, are burrowing animals.'

It is interesting to note that the common opossum (*Didelphis marsupialis*), when adult, is extremely resistant to infection either by bite or inoculation, but air-borne transmission has been successful.

Latent infection

Transmission of the rabies virus may be followed by latent infection; the disease possibly not appearing unless or until stress acts as a trigger mechanism. In bats, the virus may remain in a passive state in the brown shoulder fat, which serves as body fuel during hibernation. Dr D. G. Constantine has suggested that arousal from hibernation, or migration, may result in such stress.

A special feature of transmission of infection to vampire bats is that in feeding on infected animals they are, to quote Mr Irvine's summary of Drs Fischman and Ward's findings,

> likely to be exposed frequently to low levels of virus in the blood—conditions ideal for the establishment of a carrier state. Such a mechanism would also favour the modification of virus which appears to have taken place in bats.

A carrier state, in which no symptoms are shown but the

rabies virus is present in the animal's body, may occur not only in bats but also in Arctic foxes and in dogs affected with the Oulou fato type of rabies of Africa.

The possibility of a latent infection in foxes in Europe and the USA has been investigated, but Professor Tierkel (1959) concluded that the fox was unable to transmit the disease as a symptomless carrier, since salivary glands were never found infected without concurrent infection of the central nervous system. The *WHO Chronicle* for June 1971 commented: 'Results obtained so far suggest that the salivary excretion of rabies virus by apparently healthy foxes (indicating a carrier state), if indeed it occurs at all, has no epidemiological significance.'

A paper in *Nature*, 1969, referred to reports in Russia that people had been bitten by apparently healthy dogs and had subsequently died of rabies. A similar occurrence in India has already been referred to in Chapter 3.

The same paper in *Nature* mentioned a report that virulent virus used to challenge vaccinated dogs can be demonstrated in the saliva and urine of resistant animals for up to fourteen days after inoculation. This would imply that a dog, vaccinated in the ordinary way, could transmit infection to its owner, other people, or other animals for a short period after being itself bitten by a rabid animal.

If this were the case, dog vaccination would represent a public health hazard, admittedly small, which would have to be weighed against the public health advantages of dog vaccination. However, Dr Martin Kaplan referred (1971) to 'the completely unfounded belief that vaccination can create silent carriers and shedders of virus'. The belief, he said, originated partly from a paper by Bindrich & Schmidt (1958) which has since been challenged on the grounds that the shed virus was not, in fact, the rabies virus. Dr Kaplan added: 'Serious attempts have been made to repeat those results, but without success. All laboratory and field evidence refutes the thesis.'

Professor Steck told me: 'Among millions of vaccinated dogs there is no evidence that they can become shedders of virus after exposure to street virus without showing signs of clinical rabies.'

Vaccine-induced rabies?

Although there is at present no certain method of differentiating between street rabies and vaccine-induced rabies, United States authorities believe that it was possibly the latter which led to a pet skunk biting its owners in Yakima, Washington, in 1969. 'The interval between vaccination and onset of illness is compatible with vaccine-induced rabies.'

The animal had been vaccinated on July 29, bit its owners on August 2, was noticeably irritable on August 11, and suffered extensive paralysis and convulsions on August 12, dying on August 17. An unsuitable vaccine had been used—one recommended only for domestic animals.

Transmission by insects?

Can rabies ever be transmitted to mammals or birds by insects? Or by ticks or mites? At the time of writing there is no evidence that it can, despite some experiments designed with this possibility in mind. However, Dr R. L. Reagan and others recovered the virus in an active state after it had been harboured in ticks (*Ornithodoros turicata*) for up to a week, after feeding on the blood of bats (*Myotis lucifugus*). The virus is also reported to have been recovered from leeches and beetles in Russia. Could dung-beetles, a favourite food of the yellow mongoose, perhaps transmit the virus from carcase to mongoose?

LABORATORY DIAGNOSIS

Since the first description of them by Negri (of the University of Pavia, Italy) in 1903, the finding in brain cells of the inclusion bodies named after him has constituted the classical laboratory method of diagnosing rabies.

The technique involves staining impression smears of the cut surface of the brain (especially Ammon's horn in the hippocampal region of the cerebrum, and also in the Purkinje cells of the cerebellum) with Seller's stain, and then examining these under the microscope for the presence of Negri bodies.

The latter have to be differentiated from other inclusion bodies. In the dog and fox, for example, it is necessary to distinguish between Negri bodies, indicating rabies, and other inclusion bodies resulting from infection with canine distemper or Rubarth's disease (canine virus hepatitis/fox encephalitis). Negri bodies have a matrix which stains with eosin, with virus particles (staining blue) frequently embedded in it. Non-rabies inclusion bodies, to quote Professor Tierkel, 'lack an internal structure, have a homogeneous or smooth matrix, are highly refractile and pinker.'

Negri bodies are not invariably present in cases of rabies, and are less likely to be present if the animal is killed rather than left to die naturally of the disease. For this reason, euthanasia of dogs and cats was discouraged, owing to the great importance of an early confirmation of diagnosis.

Negri bodies may be absent in some forms of rabies, such as that occurring among foxes within the Arctic Circle. If they are present, they may be few in number and are not always typical.

Fluorescent-antibody test

In many countries the search for Negri bodies is now regarded as a somewhat unreliable method, and there is preference for the fluorescent-antibody technique. Indeed, in several countries—if not most—the latter is the principal method used nowadays as a routine test. It is a direct fluorescent reaction with acetone-fixed thin brain smears and commercial fluorescein-labelled antirabies globulin from a horse, in the presence of ultra-violet light. (See page 34.)

The fluorescent-antibody test, developed and described in 1958 by the late Dr Goldwasser and Dr Kissling, of the Communicable Disease Center, Montgomery, Alabama, has been increasingly used throughout the world. It is regarded as an accurate test and it is quick—the result can be telephoned to the patient's doctor the same day that the specimen is received.

In most countries, reliance is not placed upon a single test, and the modern practice is to confirm the fluorescent-antibody test by means of mouse inoculation. It is usual to inoculate three to five mice (preferably just weaned) intracerebrally with a brain suspension, and a similar batch with a salivary gland suspension. Symptoms, notably a staggering gait, may be observed within six to fourteen days, and the diagnosis of rabies is confirmed by the fluorescent-antibody test (or the demonstration of Negri bodies in the mouse brains). For a negative result (ie confirmation that rabies is *not* present) it is necessary to wait twenty-one days.

The corneal test

In 1969 Dr L. G. Schneider described a diagnostic test which could be applied to the living animal shedding rabies virus in its saliva. The basis of the test is that infection of the eye apparently coincides with infection of the salivary glands. The test involves pressing a clean glass slid against the eyeball. This procedure, it is stated, may be repeated several days in succession without harm to the animal's eye. The slide collects cells from the cornea which are then fixed and treated with fluorescent antibody before being examined under the microscope, in the presence of ultra-violet light. The result is considered positive when one or more infected cells are present, and Dr Schneider examines 700-800 cells before recording a negative result.

Experimentally it was found that rabies could be diagnosed before the onset of clinical symptoms in 70 per cent of infected mice in the laboratory. In all fatal cases, Dr Schneider reported, the test gave a positive result before death.

This test confirmed the diagnosis of rabies in a girl patient in Mexico, and doubtless in many other cases. However, to quote the Waterhouse Committee report, 'the test is not very reliable in dogs, and even less so in large animals'. Professor Steck commented: 'It is not used in Switzerland. It is useful as an experimental tool, but is not as reliable as the fluorescent-antibody test of brain material.'

Chapter Six

Control Measures

It is interesting to note that rabies was eradicated from the Scandinavian countries, by the elimination of stray dogs and the enforcement of quarantine measures, as early as 1826—long before the nature of the causal agent of rabies was even partially understood; in fact when Louis Pasteur was only four years old.

In 1875 the Prussian government introduced legislation requiring the killing of all dogs suspected of being rabid, and also requiring that all dogs in a district where there had been an outbreak should be kept on a leash and muzzled when allowed out-of-doors.

There was much opposition by dog-owners to the local muzzling orders introduced in Britain during the nineteenth century, but eventually rabies was made a notifiable disease in 1886, and stringent control measures were eventually applied throughout the country. One of the measures taken involved the destruction of numerous stray dogs then roaming at will.

Elimination of strays

This measure, which remains an essential part of modern

rabies control programmes, is easier to consider in theory than to carry out in practice; and in the past somewhat macabre techniques have sometimes been employed. For example, the report of the Singapore municipality for 1888 includes the following passage on the subject of stray dogs:

> They are caught by means of long tongs or nippers and put into an iron cage on wheels, which is drawn by a bullock. The cart is divided into two compartments, one for dogs likely to be claimed, the other for those which from their appearance have no master. After the morning work the cage is taken to the pound at the Ord Road Police Station. The good dogs in the one compartment are taken out and pounded, while the cage with the others is detached from its wheels, lifted up by a crane and dropped into the river at high-water. Three minutes are then allowed for the dogs to be in the water, when the cage is again lifted, re-attached to its wheels, and the carcases carried out to Geylang for the purpose of burial. A very large number of dogs exist in Singapore which really have no master, living a wandering life without any certain subsistence and, of course, when seen abroad have no registered number and collar. It is this class which is so dangerous, and the only method of dealing with them is utter destruction. Unless this is done there will be no safety.

Two or three years later muzzling was enforced, and this, together with the prohibition of the importation of dogs into the island, achieved what the 1888 dog tax and issue of badges for registered dogs had begun. Rabies was eradicated from Singapore by 1892.

In India, at Rawalpindi, during the 1939-45 war, two Alsatians were used by the Army in the difficult task of rounding up stray dogs, as part of the anti-rabies campaign there. Warning notices were issued to dog-owners, telling them to keep

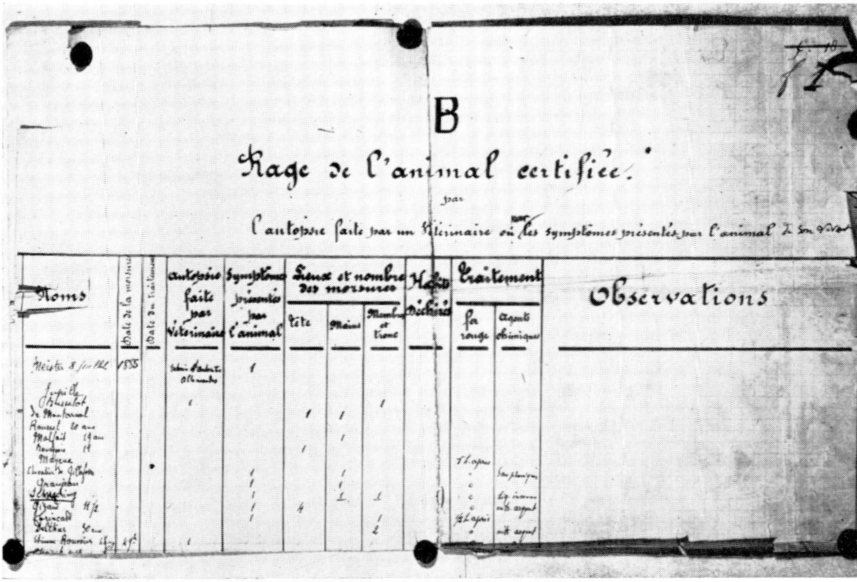
B

Rage de l'animal certifiée

par

l'autopsie faite par un Vétérinaire ou par les symptômes présentés par l'animal

Noms	Date de la morsure	Date du traitement	Autopsie faite par Vétérinaire	Symptômes présentés par l'animal	Lieux et nombre des morsures: Tête	Mains	Membres et tronc	Habits déchirés	Traitement: fer rouge	agents chimiques	Observations
Meister 8 [illegible]	1885		[illegible] Allemands	1							

Page 103 (*above*) A historic document: a rabies certificate bearing the name of Joseph Meister, the first patient to be treated with rabies vaccine after being bitten; (*below*) bitten people and their relatives at Pasteur's laboratory in the Rue d'Ulm, Paris, 1885. Pasteur is on the left; Dr Grancher (right) is treating a patient

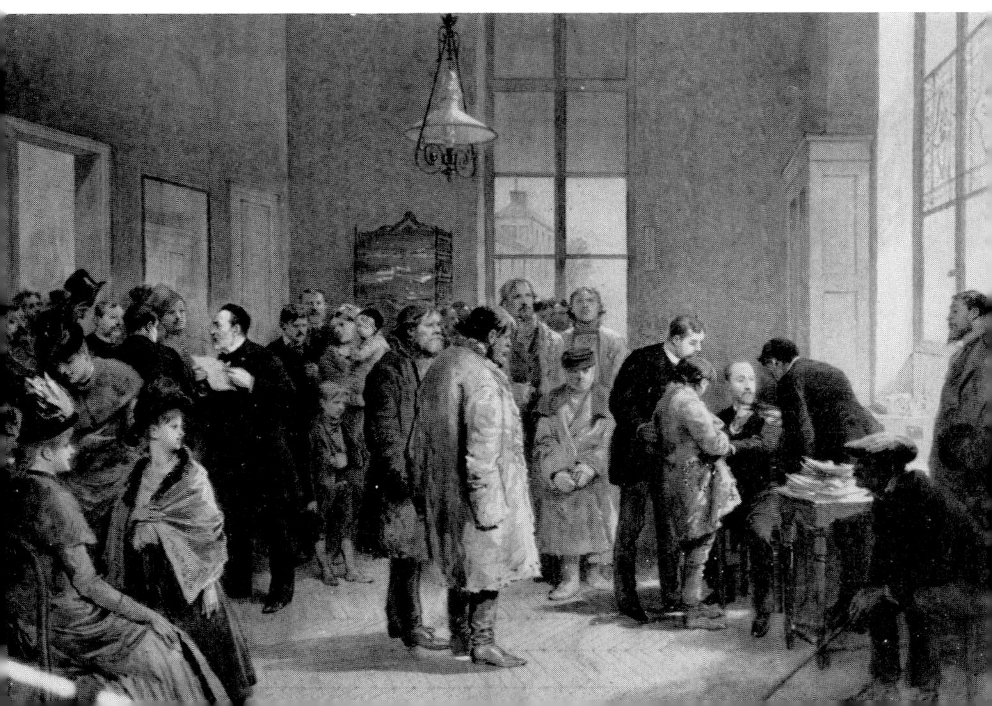

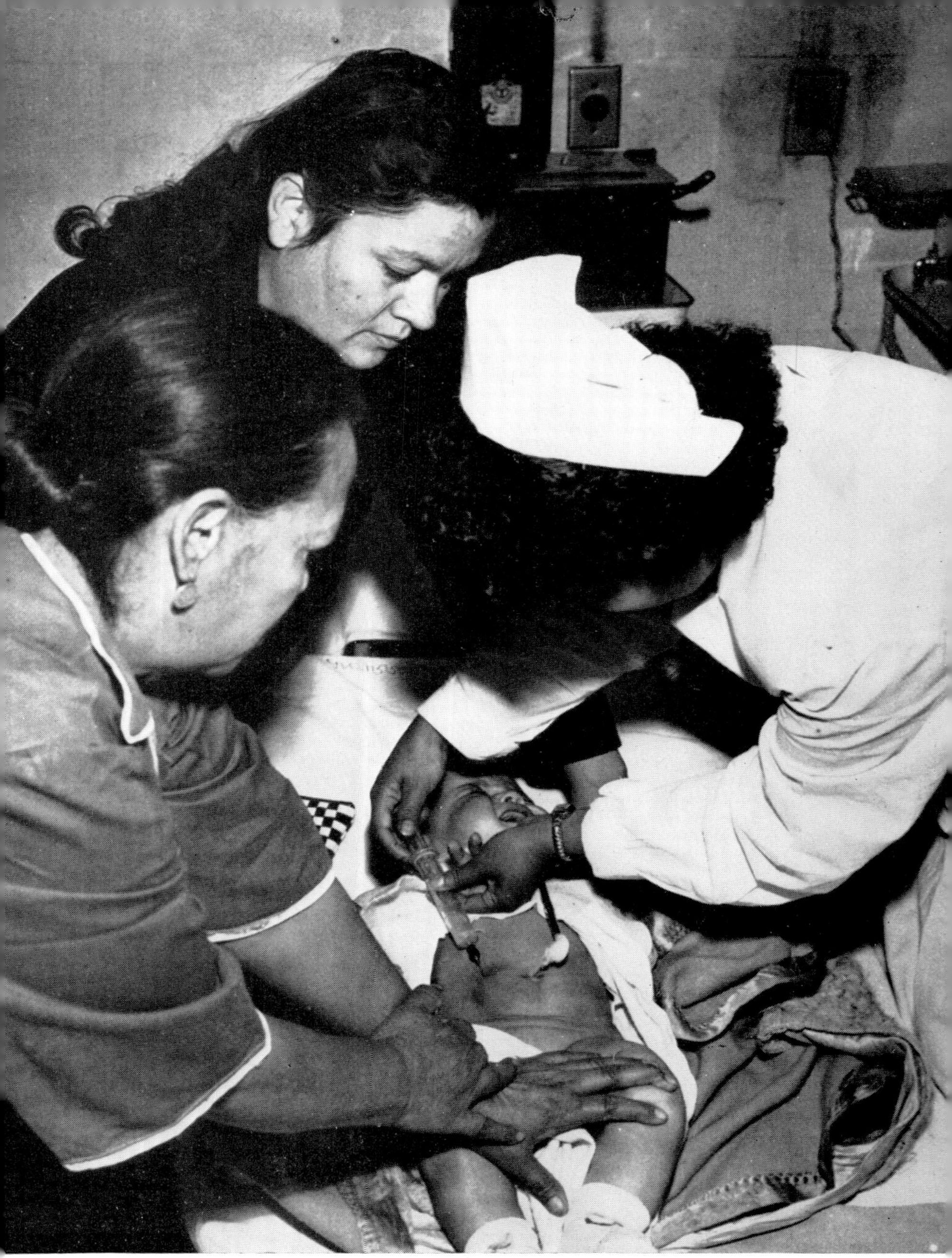

Page 104 One of at least fourteen injections of vaccine for a child bitten by a rabid animal

their dogs indoors at a certain time. After this warning, the Alsatians would come barking and gambolling among the dogs still at liberty, and would lead as many as forty or fifty to an Army shooting range. All dogs would enter by the same door; but the two Alsatians would immediately pass through another doorway opposite, when the door would quickly be shut behind them. The strays, which they had tricked into following them, would then be shot. It was, in practice, a humane way of dealing with the problem of collecting strays. As to the 'treachery' of the Alsatians, one can only say that there have been so-called Judas sheep, and at least one Judas cow, employed to lure their fellow creatures into slaughter-houses; and perhaps it is inevitable that there should have been Judas dogs such as these.

Syringe and gun

If Britain was somewhat tardy in ridding herself of rabies, her overseas veterinary services were energetic in their efforts to control the disease in many parts of the world where British rule or administration prevailed.

In the Federation of Malaya, where animal health had deteriorated during the war-time occupation by the Japanese, rabies had become firmly established in the northern half of the Federation, and in 1952 it spread to the capital, Kuala Lumpur. This town, which had been free of rabies for twenty-one years, now had a dog population estimated at 20,000, including a high proportion of ownerless strays. Conditions favoured the spread of the disease, and cases were numerous. Availability of the Flury strain chick-embryo-adapted vaccine encouraged the idea for a compulsory vaccination programme. This was carried out with public support, and by the end of the year nearly 18,000 dogs had been vaccinated and over 12,000 destroyed in and around Kuala Lumpur. Whereas there had been thirty-five cases of rabies in July, there were none in December.

Encouraged by this success, the veterinary department carried out a programme of vaccination in all affected States in the following year. Again public support was forthcoming, and nearly 74,000 dogs were vaccinated; unvaccinated, ownerless strays being destroyed. Mr W. E. Lancaster, CBE, MA, MRCVS, commented:

> This policy of attacking the disease with a syringe in one hand and a gun in the other proved so successful that no case of rabies was detected in any part of the Federation after June 1953. . . . In order to consolidate the victory, vaccination was carried out over the whole Federation in 1954; 115,000 dogs were vaccinated and 30,000 destroyed. For the first time in memory it was possible to remove all rabies restrictions, allow free movement of dogs within the Federation, and amend the regulations for the entry of dogs into the country.

Contraceptives and rabies

In some countries the killing of stray dogs is not an acceptable rabies-control measure for religious reasons. This is true of Thailand where, in 1963, fifty people died from rabies in Bangkok alone. In the villages many ownerless dogs run wild in packs, and add to the rabies risk. Moreover, these animals multiply at an alarming rate.

Accordingly a Thai-American university team carried out a pilot trial with a contraceptive drug among sixty bitches of two villages in the northern part of the country.

These sixty bitches all had owners but were free-roaming, and they were selected on the basis that each had had at least one litter of puppies. All were vaccinated against rabies, and every other one received an injection of medrxyprogesteroneacetate. This proved to be 81 per cent effective in preventing reproduction, and Dr Chamroon Yasmuth and his colleagues reported: 'Villagers whose dogs were in the test group were happy with the contraceptive effect of the drug, especially as an approach to the rabies problem, and their dogs appeared fat and healthy.'

Further studies are being made into this promising method of reducing the dog population in areas where rabies is rife.

Dog vaccination in the USA

Page 42 shows the remarkable reduction in the incidence of rabies in dogs which has been achieved, despite a growing wildlife rabies problem, in the USA.

Publicity campaigns to inform the public about the disease, stray-dog control, and mass vaccination of dogs have all contributed to success.

In 1946, when there were about twelve million dogs in the USA, there were 8,384 confirmed cases of rabies in dogs. In 1965, with an estimated dog population of 22,900,000 there were only 412 cases. In 1970 the figure was down to 185.

When a serious outbreak of wildlife rabies occurs in the USA, the Department of Public Health and/or Agriculture may call on the State Game and Fish Department to take measures to control the outbreak. Under the guidance of biologists, if possible, selective animal population reductions will then be effected in the area. The aim is to reduce the contact rate between infected and susceptible animals, by the only means at present available: trapping, shooting, gassing or use of poisoned baits. This was first carried out in the coyote-rabies outbreaks which occurred in California and Nevada in 1915-20.

Eggs containing 1ml of a 10 per cent solution of strychnine in honey-water have been used in Ohio in an attempt to reduce the number of skunks during an outbreak of rabies among these animals. The incidence of the disease was successfully lessened, and according to reports no domestic animals or persons were accidentally poisoned during the entire campaign.

Findings in the eastern part of the USA suggest that a population density of one fox per sq km will maintain a rabies epizootic. In order to interrupt the spread of the disease among foxes, it is necessary to reduce their numbers until there is one fox or less per five sq km.

A Canadian campaign

The successful application of measures drastically to reduce the incidence of wildlife rabies in the province of Alberta, Canada, during the serious 1952-4 outbreak there has been described by the two veterinarians who advised on the campaign throughout (Dr E. E. Ballantyne and Dr J. G. O'Donoghue).

As Alberta is three times the size of the British Isles and five times the size of New York State, the scale of operations and the distances involved are perhaps difficult to visualise for those living in smallish countries; but the fact that heads of animals believed to be rabid had to be sent anything up to 900 miles for laboratory examination gives some idea of the practical difficulties.

The inhabitants of Alberta were not familiar with rabies which spread, it seems, from the North-West Territory, where it had been endemic for many years. The disease was apparently brought by foxes migrating southwards.

Four dogs were bitten by a red fox which made its way into the village of Fort Fitzgerald, and three of them died of rabies about a fortnight later. Elsewhere another dog was attacked by a fox, and in the farming district of Fort Vermilion several pigs were attacked by a rabid wolf. In this and another similar farming area, a total of 80 head of cattle, 150 pigs, and 25 horses died of rabies. Rabid foxes caused the largest proportion of deaths, but many resulted from wolf bites.

Wild animals involved in the epidemic included, besides foxes and wolves, the following species: bear, beaver, coyote, lynx, moose, rabbit, and weasel.

Altogether some 200 people had to undergo a course of anti-rabies inoculations, following bites from dogs or cats; exposure through skinning wild animals with ungloved hands; scratches from rabid lynx; bites from mice suspected of being rabid; and exposure during the handling of farm livestock later known to be rabid.

Reports on the advance of the disease in the forests of northern Alberta were gathered from forest rangers, registered trappers, and members of the Royal Canadian Mounted Police. These, collated, enabled a very good picture of the rabies situation to be obtained by the authorities.

Control measures were accompanied by a province-wide campaign to inform members of the general public on the nature and dangers of rabies, and the measures and precautions necessary to reduce its spread and, if possible, eradicate it.

Local byelaws were passed throughout the province requiring that stray dogs be destroyed and others kept tied up. Some non-strays were put down because their owners preferred not to see them miserable as a result of being perpetually on a chain. On several Indian reservations there was imposed a limitation of dogs to two per person, unless more were needed for sledge teams.

Compulsory vaccination of all dogs north of the 55th parallel was undertaken in 1952-3, with revaccination in the autumn of 1953. South of the line, vaccination was left to the owner's discretion, and had to be paid for privately.

Dog vaccination is accepted as a cardinal principle in wildlife rabies control, since dogs can otherwise so readily act as carriers of the infection between wild animals and man, and wild animals and farm livestock; besides occasionally transmitting the infection back to wildlife.

A law making the fox a protected animal was repealed or suspended, and professional trappers were employed drastically to reduce the numbers of foxes, wolves, and coyotes. Poisoned baits, snares, and traps were all used. Early in the second year of the epidemic some 5,000 miles of traplines were in existence.

The trappers mostly remained in the forests for weeks on end, with temperatures sometimes as low as −50°F, except for the monthly collection of supplies. Every sort of transport was used in winter—dog teams, dogs with panniers, horses, and motor vehicles where the trappers were working not far from roads. In summer, horses and canoes carried trappers and their equipment.

Apart from the main body of trappers, which at the peak period totalled 150, some 15 were assigned to the duty of reducing the number of wolves, coyotes, and cougars in the forests on the eastern slopes of the Rocky Mountains.

At the beginning of the campaign, both cyanide and strychnine were used as poisons for baits; but later the use of cyanide was abandoned except in coyote guns. In winter, baits were usually made up of lard or other animal fat, with cubes or pellets of strychnine inside, and a feather attached to attract the animal. In summer, beef fat or a mixture of lard and beeswax, or similar preparations suited to a higher temperature, were preferred.

Strychnine pellets were sometimes enclosed in moose skin, or mixed with the marrow and put in bones. Wolves were also enticed by a draw-bait consisting of the carcase of a horse, cow, or rabbit, with poisoned baits put out all round some inches deep in the snow where they would be inaccessible to birds. Another effective bait for wolves, coyotes, and foxes was made by boiling an egg for two minutes, inserting strychnine, and covering the hole with adhesive tape. Canned dog food was another bait. Against lynx, several of which became rabid, leading to at least one attack on children, squirrel meat was the bait of choice.

Many wolves were killed on the surface of frozen lakes, on which they tend to foregather when there is deep snow.

In summer, trapping was largely abandoned; the men searching for animals' dens, often 40-70 miles deep inside the forests.

Cyanide guns were introduced for use against coyotes, and some 30,000 of these weapons were supplied, many to farmers when coyotes began invading agricultural land. The gun killed the coyote by ejecting cyanide into its mouth when a ·38 cartridge was fired by means of a trigger mechanism, actuated when the animal took the bait.

According to reliable estimates the kill, in all forest areas from October 1952 to March 1954, included: 50,000 foxes; 35,000 coyotes; 7,500 lynx; 1,850 bears; 500 skunks; and 64 cougars (pumas); also 4,000 wolves.

The campaign had a successful outcome, in the sense that rabies disappeared from the province, and remained absent for several years. Without such drastic measures, rabies might have become endemic in Alberta.

Nevertheless, the figures may bring a frown to many conservationists; while other people may shudder at the thought of the extent of animal suffering caused by traps and snares and strychnine. One can only say that rabies, too, can mean an unpleasant death, and that in the interests of men, women and children—not to mention farm livestock and domestic pets—this campaign was considered essential. Moreover, moose and deer increased.

Control measures in Europe

Poisoning has been resorted to in Europe, and may be the only economically feasible method in sparsely populated areas; but it requires the services of sufficient experienced trappers with first-hand knowledge of the habits of foxes and other animals, and it offends public opinion in many countries. Where it has been adopted, poisons have included cyanide, strychnine, and sodium fluoroacetate ('compound 1080').

Public opinion has likewise been against trapping and snaring in several countries, though these methods are considered more efficient than shooting if they are applied during autumn and winter—the time of year when foxes are chiefly on the move. Even where the climate of opinion is favourable to such methods, there may not be enough skilled trappers to implement them.

During the setting of traps, gloves—which are kept for this purpose only—must be worn. Rotten fish or fox urine is used to attract foxes to the trapping site.

European experience bears out American experience, in that although trapping ahead of a rabies outbreak appears to be the right thing to do, it is not always possible to raise the necessary funds or to obtain the co-operation of the public before rabies is a reality in their immediate vicinity.

Shooting of foxes can be carried out on a voluntary basis by amateurs, perhaps encouraged by a bounty payable on each fox killed; or it can be undertaken, wholly or in part, by professionals. Various proprietary devices which simulate rabbit distress cries may be used to bring foxes within shooting range. Such calls, it was recommended, should be used late in the day and especially on days with a low wind velocity.

Shooting is one of the two methods which finds favour in many European countries; the other is gassing. The latter can be very effective in reducing fox populations if it is carried out at the proper time, ie when the vixen stays with her cubs during the first three weeks at least.

The poison gases used are prussic acid and hydrophosphoric acid; the necessary chemicals being introduced into fox earths (and badger setts) by pumping or by means of long-handled shovels. In the presence of moisture and carbon dioxide the gas is released and permeates below ground; the entrances and exits having been closed.

'Cymag' is a convenient cyanide preparation for this purpose, and it would appear to be humane in its action. Although death from cyanide poisoning is an unpleasant one to witness —dogs have convulsions and utter a cry—accidents which have involved two men in England (one using 'Cymag' and the other using liquid hydrocyanic acid) suggests that no suffering is caused owing to rapid loss of consciousness. Fortunately, the two men lived to tell the tale!

A Danish campaign

Dr J. Muller, of the State Veterinary Serum Laboratory, Copenhagen, from whose paper given at the WHO conference at Frankfurt-on-Main in 1968, I have—with his permission—abstracted, described there a campaign against wildlife rabies carried out in Denmark. The infection had spread across the Danish-German frontier at the beginning of 1964, and moved northwards in two waves until it was stopped 30km from the border in August 1965. Two methods of control were practised. Shooting, encouraged by the payment of a bounty on all foxes killed, was carried out within a zone 60-70km deep; and gassing within a 30-70km zone north of the frontier was supervised by local police officers having a personal knowledge of wildlife.

According to estimates by Danish wildlife biologists, who co-operated in the fox population reduction, shooting as the sole method of control resulted in a 25 per cent kill; while shooting and gassing combined resulted in an 80 per cent reduction.

After the disappearance of rabies from this area, measures to maintain the fox population at a substantially reduced level were maintained. For this purpose, shooting was preferred to gassing.

Danish experience has confirmed the American finding that one fox per 5sq km is, from the rabies control point of view, the permissible maximum.

Future possibilities

Two other methods of fox control are in the experimental stage. One involves the use of a hormone, such as stilboestrol, to bring about infertility; the other is fox vaccination. Foxes can be successfully immunised against rabies with only a 3ml dose of a suitable vaccine. The problem with both methods, of course, is one of administration. Giving vaccine by mouth in some form of bait, and the use of automatic devices, are among the possibilities that have been considered.

Other control measures

In *Denmark* all dogs in South Jutland have to be vaccinated every three years with the ERA vaccine produced by the Connaught Medical Research Laboratories, Toronto. This is a live vaccine of pig tissue-culture origin. Both the cost of the vaccination and the vaccination fee are paid for by the Danish government, so that there is no charge to the dog-owner. The vaccination of cats remains on a voluntary basis.

If an outbreak of rabies occurs among dogs or cats, an area (of 2km or more radius) is declared in which dogs and cats must be kept indoors for three months, except while being exercised on a leash. All stray dogs and cats found away from buildings are liable to be shot. All known contacts of rabid animals are immediately destroyed, even if vaccinated; the exception being cattle and horses which may be kept if certain conditions are observed.

In *France* there is provision for movement control, leashing of dogs, and compulsory vaccination to be ordered in any area where an isolated outbreak of rabies occurs. In practice, vaccination has in the past been voluntary and in order to encourage it, new regulations were expected in 1971 to allow a vaccinated dog to be kept (if under veterinary surveillance and restriction) after contact with a rabid animal, instead of having to be destroyed.

In the Federal Republic of *Germany* a 'danger area' is declared when rabies has been detected, and the public are informed accordingly; with notices displayed at the roadside, railway stations, ports, etc. If wildlife is involved, the prescribed area may be of 10km radius; where a dog or cat is involved the size of the area is determined by local circumstances. Within the area all dogs must be kept on a leash, and cats kept under strict control. Dogs and cats found wandering are impounded if practicable; otherwise shot. In-contact and bitten dogs and cats may be destroyed. Farm and 'zoo' animals may be destroyed or isolated. Where an animal has died of rabies (or been slaughtered on account of the disease) disinfection of the premises must be carried out; articles such as collars and muzzles being burnt.

In *Switzerland* the control of rabies is complicated by the exigencies of tourism. Tourists bring dogs and cats with them. These must have been vaccinated not less than thirty days or more than one year previously. The indigenous dogs (some 160,000) must be vaccinated every year with an inactivated vaccine, or every two years with a live vaccine.

In a declared infected zone, dogs and cats must be either

confined to a building or tied up in an enclosed area; the alternative being destruction. All domestic animals bitten by a rabid animal must normally be destroyed; but if already vaccinated, permission may be obtained to keep them subject to re-vaccination and thirty days' quarantine. The latter requirement is also applied to unvaccinated domestic animals in contact with, but not bitten by, rabid animals.

In areas where rabies has been confirmed among wildlife but not among domestic animals, dogs must be muzzled and exercised on a leash.

The man in charge

The report of WHO's expert committee on rabies, 1966, states that experience has shown the desirability of placing any nation-wide control programme in the hands of a public health veterinarian, given full executive powers and devoting all his working hours to this sole task.

As a co-ordinator he is responsible for:

(1) working closely with committees of medical and veterinary men in circulating information on current control methods;

(2) enlisting the support of livestock organisations, animal welfare societies, kennel clubs, and sportsmen's clubs;

(3) arranging regular exchanges of information with officials in other countries;

(4) collecting and analysing data relating to animal bites, exposure to infection by other means in human beings, cases of rabies, use of vaccines and their side-effects;

(5) developing and improving reporting systems and the interpretation of findings in close collaboration with diagnostic laboratories, and providing information on the geographical movement of infection throughout his country;

(6) improving methods for the despatch of specimens to laboratories;

(7) conducting training courses and organising research into various aspects of rabies control; and

(8) promoting a continuous and energetic publicity campaign to keep the general public informed about the disease.

Travel and trade

Rabies control measures may be severely tested, and require more manpower to enforce and more expenditure of money to maintain, when dogs, cats, exotic pets, and laboratory animals are moved from country to country in ever-growing numbers.

Against a background of increased air traffic, and a flourishing international trade in pedigree dogs and cats, imports of these creatures have risen steeply in many countries. For example, in 1949 approximately 1,800 dogs and 100 cats entered Britain. In 1969 the figures were over 4,000 and 1,000 respectively; and 76 per cent of them arrived by air.

With more people taking their holidays abroad now, with more cars on the roads and on the ferries, some countries, eg Switzerland, have their native dog populations considerably increased by the dogs of holiday-makers. So far as the control of rabies is concerned, tourism does add to the problems. So do political refugees, as Uganda found in the 1960s.

Quarantine

An important rabies control measure, adopted by many countries throughout the world, is the requirement of a period of isolation in State-owned or officially approved quarantine kennels for imported dogs and cats.

In countries where rabies is endemic, quarantine restrictions are not usually considered worthwhile; though vaccination may be required as a condition of entry.

Control Measures

In countries where rabies is not endemic—occurring neither among dogs nor wildlife—quarantine is commonly but not universally applied, and constitutes a valuable and often permanent method of defence against the introduction of the disease.

The idea behind quarantine is, of course, that if the animal is going to become rabid the disease will show itself before the expiration of the quarantine period, while the animal is still in isolation under veterinary supervision, and not constituting a hazard to the public.

The length of quarantine decided upon is in the nature of a compromise; the authorities taking into account not so much the longest known incubation period of rabies as the commonly occurring incubation periods. Other factors which may enter into the decision are the cost of maintaining quarantine kennels (if State-owned), any hardship to owner or animal felt to be inflicted by a long period of quarantine, and the realisation that too long a period is likely to encourage the smuggling of pet animals in order to avoid quarantine altogether.

Smuggling of dogs (or cats) into a country can lead to very serious consequences. It led, almost certainly, to the re-introduction of rabies into Britain in 1918, resulting in 318 cases, and taking four years to eradicate again. In the Netherlands, in 1962, one if not two smuggled dogs apparently led to an outbreak of rabies among household pets in Amsterdam which cost the lives of five people.

Except for a temporary lengthening of the quarantine period in 1970, and a reduction to four months during the 1914-18 war, Britain has always required six months' quarantine. Visitors, and sometimes returning expatriates, have often protested over this period, which must seem very long to a dog and can prove costly to the owner. Yet six months is not an absurdly long time, as writers of letters to newspapers often assert.

The fifth report of the WHO Expert Committee on Rabies recommended:

> Countries now free of rabies should continue either to prohibit the importation of dogs and cats or to subject them to a prolonged period of quarantine, preferably four or more months, at the port of entry. If the period of quarantine is only four months, leashing and surveillance for an additional two months are recommended.

Denmark, Eire, Finland, the Netherlands and Norway are among countries which either do, or have in the past, required six months' quarantine.

Four months' quarantine is required by Iceland, and now by Norway (which adds two months' local restriction at the animal's destination), and by Sweden (if the dog is from a country where rabies is endemic).

Australia and New Zealand will admit dogs only from each other's territory or from Britain. Canada applies 90 days' quarantine to any dog coming from a territory where rabies is present, but makes an exception to the rule in the case of the USA.

All dogs, cats, and monkeys imported into the USA must be inspected by the quarantine officer at the port of arrival. Dogs must have been vaccinated against rabies unless under three months old, or unless they have been for the last six months in a rabies-free country, or unless destined for a zoological park or research establishment, or a wild member of the dog family (when six months' isolation will be required).

Vaccination before, or on, arrival is required by several countries, and in the former case a certificate will be necessary; and the vaccination must have been carried out within certain stipulated time limits. These vary in accordance with national regulations. (The latter are altered from time to time, and it is important that the latest position is ascertained well in advance of the journey.)

Import licences are required for dogs or cats to be sent or taken to Britain, and must be obtained in advance. The applicant is provided with information about the quarantine regulations, together with a list of approved quarantine kennels (there were 46 of these in 1971) and approved carriers authorised to transport animals from place of entry to the kennels. On receipt of a completed application form, and before issuing a licence, the authorities check that a place in quarantine kennels has, in fact, been reserved for the animal, and that transport has been arranged.

Management of quarantine kennels

The design and management of quarantine premises are almost as important as the period of isolation itself. Bad design and layout of buildings, under-staffing, a faulty routine, a lack of cleanliness, or the leaving open by mistake of a gate for only a moment or two—any one of these factors could lead to one dog (or cat) infecting another before symptoms of rabies had appeared or been recognised.

It is now believed that the dog Fritz (referred to in Chapter 3) which became rabid shortly after release from six months' quarantine, had become infected not in Germany but inside the quarantine kennels, where a collie from India had died of rabies in the preceding July, and where a third dog, Whiskey (also from Germany) became rabid during the month following Fritz's release.

These three incidents, taken together, seemed highly suspicious, and an official enquiry was conducted by two distinguished veterinarians. They concluded, in their final report, that infection had been transmitted ('by direct or indirect means') within the kennels from the collie to Fritz, and possibly also to Whiskey. As a result, government approval of these kennels for quarantine purposes was withdrawn.

Subsequently, detailed recommendations were made by the Waterhouse Committee for improving the design and operation of quarantine kennels, in order to minimise this risk of infection being transferred from one animal inmate to another. They also recommended that quarantine should be supplemented by vaccination, as a further precaution, and this has since become the rule in Britain.

The operation of quarantine premises, whether in State or private ownership, is certainly no sinecure. The veterinarian in charge, and the kennelmaids or other staff, need to be constantly on the alert for the first symptoms of rabies; and they should themselves be vaccinated against the disease, for their own protection.

Naturally, other health problems besides rabies will arise from time to time. In one country, infestation of the buildings with tropical ticks (brought with them by imported dogs) assumed serious proportions.

INTERNATIONAL CO-OPERATION

Although rabies control programmes are nowadays mostly national in so far as their direction is concerned, the efforts of the World Health Organisation and of individual rabies experts have made international co-operation a reality, with exchange of information, meetings of delegates to discuss new techniques and discoveries, and even the establishment of regional centres. For example, the Pan American Zoonoses Centre in Buenos Aires, Argentina, initiated a rabies surveillance programme for the Americas in 1969.

In Europe, to take another example, a research programme was drawn up in 1969 by a group of advisers from several countries, convened jointly by the Food and Agriculture Organisation of the United Nations and by the World Health

Organisation. Research teams from Czechoslovakia, the Netherlands, Switzerland, and West Germany participated. The main objective was to determine whether wildlife rabies in central Europe could be eradicated, and whether this could be done by the control of fox populations without upsetting too greatly the ecological balance of other species. Nine test areas in co-operating countries were selected. The importance of rodents and bats, and the question of symptomless carriers of rabies, were among subjects selected for investigation.

Chapter Seven

Rabies Vaccines

Vaccination against rabies stems from the famous work carried out in the 1880s by Louis Pasteur, in collaboration with Pierre Roux and Charles Chamberland.

Pasteur demonstrated that the infective agent—called virus after the Latin word for poison—was present and multiplied in the brain and spinal cord of infected animals. He also showed that if infective material were inoculated into the brains of a series of rabbits, the virus became more virulent for rabbits at each passage, while the incubation period of the disease became progressively shortened from the usual fifteen days to seven days. He called this virus 'fixed' to distinguish it from the 'street' virus causing natural infection in dogs.

By passage of the street virus through a series of ninety or a hundred rabbits, he produced a fixed virus which proved far less virulent for dogs. Similarly, passage of the virus through monkeys decreased the virulence of the virus for dogs and rabbits. It seemed that this process of attenuation might have a practical use.

A second method of attenuation was used when Pasteur began work on the preparation of the first anti-rabies vaccine. Fixed virus was injected into rabbits, and when these died their spinal cords were removed and pieces—a few centimetres long—detached and suspended over a desiccating agent in flasks kept at room temperature. After about a fortnight the infected material had, as a result of the drying process, lost virtually all its virulence. By having a series of flasks, with pieces of spinal cord inserted on successive days, Pasteur obtained for all practical purposes the infective agent with a progressive range of attenuation. (It should be added that some later authorities have inclined to the view that drying merely reduced the concentration of virus below the level at which it will produce rabies, without sacrificing its antigenic property.)

Fragments of infected spinal cord, removed from the flasks after drying, were then used in the preparation of a liquid which could be used for inoculation. Each day a dog received a dose of this liquid; the first dose being prepared from material which had received the longest drying period, and the last dose made from material which had been in a flask for only a day or two. By this means Pasteur found that a dog could be rendered immune to rabies, for even his most virulent virus inoculated under the skin or even into the brain did not produce the disease.

Not every dog was successfully immunised in the early work, and there were some *accidents,* to use Pasteur's own word. However, by 6 July 1885 he had fifty dogs of various breeds and ages, all successfully immunised and able to withstand a challenge dose of virulent virus. On that day a nine-year-old boy, Joseph Meister, was brought to Pasteur's laboratory. The boy had been attacked by an evidently rabid dog and severely bitten on the hand and legs. The worst of the wounds had been cauterised twelve hours after they were inflicted.

Pasteur called in for consultation Dr Jacques Grancher, a professor at the Faculty of Medicine, and another medical man. They examined the boy, found at least fourteen bite-

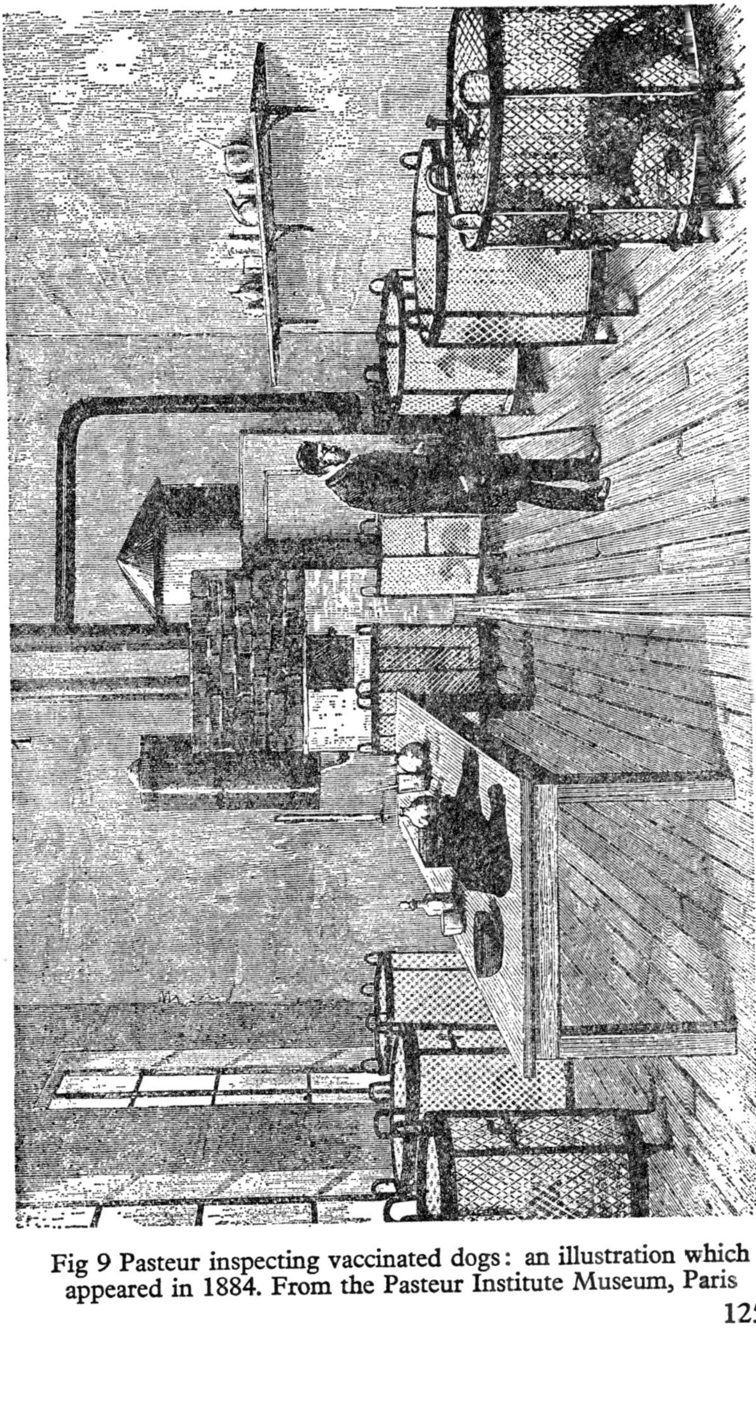

Fig 9 Pasteur inspecting vaccinated dogs: an illustration which appeared in 1884. From the Pasteur Institute Museum, Paris

wounds, and agreed that the death of the patient appeared inevitable. Pasteur told the two consultants of his most recent work on rabies vaccination and, with Grancher's support, decided—'not without keen and cruel anxiety'—to try on Joseph Meister the method that he had used with success on dogs.

On 26 October 1885 Pasteur was able to announce to the *Académie des Sciences*, Paris, that Joseph's health left nothing to be desired. The boy had escaped, he pointed out, the rabies which could have followed from the bites and also that which could have followed from the inoculation of fully virulent virus.

Pasteur also told of treatment of a fourteen-year-old shepherd boy, badly bitten when trying to save six younger boys from attack by a dog which he stunned, after freeing his left hand from its mouth, with one of his clogs. This second boy, Jean Baptiste Jupelle, had been under treatment for six days when the *Académie des Sciences* meeting was held. The president of the *Académie* observed that the session would always remain memorable in the history of medicine, and always glorious for French science.

It was indeed a triumph for Pasteur. Both boys survived (Joseph Meister was later to become a porter at the Pasteur Institute in Paris), and this method of treating people bitten by rabid animals was widely adopted and became standard practice.

Pasteur's technique of vaccine production was modified in 1908 when Fermi used phenol to attenuate the virus instead of relying on the drying of the infected spinal cords.

Semple-type vaccines

In 1919 Fermi's method was, in turn, modified by Semple, who used both phenol and a temperature of 37 °C. Semple-type vaccines have been used all over the world and have afforded good protection against the disease.

In 1935 Dr P. Lépine showed that it was preferable to substitute rabbit's (or sheep's) brain for the spinal cord used by Pasteur and by his successors.

A disadvantage of Semple-type vaccines prepared from brain or spinal cord tissue is that they may, in a small percentage of patients, give rise to serious side-effects or even death. An allergic encephalomyelitis may be caused—due, it is believed, to the myelin in the nervous tissue used in the vaccine —and if the patient recovers, he may be left with some degree of paralysis or neuritis. Complications of this kind have affected about 1 in 1,600 people treated; with 1 in 11,000 dying as a result of the vaccine treatment.

Because of these risks, Semple-type vaccines are not used for the immunisation of people likely to be exposed to rabies infection as a result of their work, but only as a means of protecting a person already bitten by a rabid animal.

Attempts have been made to overcome the danger from myelin. The Fuenzalida vaccine, first described in 1955, is prepared from mice under ten days old, before myelination has taken place. Ultra-violet light is used to inactivate the virus.

Except when some batches of this vaccine were made from older mice, there have apparently been no complications of an allergic nature; though viruses (other than rabies) present but unsuspected in the mice may constitute a risk. Fuenzalida vaccine has been widely used in man, both in South America and in Russia.

The Pasteur Institute, Paris, was in 1971 supplying large quantities of vaccine prepared from the brains of new-born mice, but inactivated with beta-propiolactone instead of ultra-violet irradiation, both for medical and veterinary use in Latin America. For human use, Russia was using a vaccine prepared from the brains of new-born rats.

In 1968 Dr G. S. Turner and Professor C. Kaplan described a method of avoiding encephalomyelitis resulting from using for vaccine production adult mammalian nerve tissue. They used Arcton, a fluorocarbon, to remove some of the harmful material. A Semple-type vaccine prepared in this way may prove valuable.

Duck-embryo vaccine

A different type of vaccine was developed by Dr H. M. Powell and Dr C. G. Culbertson, and first described by them in 1950. The rabies virus was grown in duck embryo, partially purified, and then inactivated with beta-propiolactone. This type of vaccine has the advantage that it is safer than Semple-type vaccines, which to some extent it has replaced. It is not entirely free from side-effects, however, as occasionally it gives rise to an allergy associated with duck-embryo protein; while neurological complications have been reported in one out of every 25,000 people treated with it.

Duck-embryo vaccine (often abbreviated to DEV) can be used both for the protection of people whose work carries a high risk of exposure to rabies infection, and also for treating people bitten by rabid animals. For the latter purpose it is given as the usual course of at least fourteen injections, plus booster doses; while for immunising unexposed people two injections of vaccine at 4-6 week intervals, plus a booster dose after six months, or three injections at weekly intervals plus a booster dose at three months, are given.

Dr R. K. Sikes has stated that people immunised with duck-embryo vaccine generally had a faster antibody response than those immunised with nervous-tissue vaccine. However, the antibody titre usually reached a higher level in people vaccinated with nervous-tissue vaccine.

In Britain and Russia, to name but two countries, doubts

have sometimes been expressed concerning the efficacy of duck-embryo vaccine in stimulating sufficient antibody production to give protection. Comparative vaccine experiments in animals have shown duck-embryo vaccine to be less potent in this respect than brain vaccines; while antibody levels in treated people have sometimes been disconcertingly low.

It was pointed out in *WHO Chronicle* (1971) that one of the major difficulties in treating people exposed to rabies has been this relatively small degree of antibody production stimulated by the vaccines hitherto available, and consequently the need for 'a long course of inoculations causing great discomfort and often having serious side-effects'.

The situation is changing for the better, however, and within a few years it may be possible to dispense with a course of at least fourteen injections and to protect the bitten (or otherwise exposed) person with only two or three inoculations; or possibly with only one.

Professor C. Kaplan has mentioned the possibility of adapting the rabies virus to some new host which would result in sufficient attenuation for the virus to be used live in a vaccine for human beings; with only a single dose being needed. His own work on removing harmful substances from vaccine material of nervous-tissue origin has already been referred to. Dr R. K. Sikes and others have used different methods to achieve the same end.

Tissue-culture vaccines

At present, highly purified and concentrated tissue-culture vaccines, in the development of which WHO is assisting, seem to offer the greatest prospects of success.

The first successful tissue-culture anti-rabies vaccine was developed in Canada by Dr P. Fenje, who described his method in 1960. He adapted the ERA strain of virus (obtained from a rabid dog) to hamster kidney cells.

In 1964 Dr M. K. Abelseth described the further adaptation of the ERA virus to pig's kidney cells, and the production of a live, attenuated vaccine. This has been used with great success for dogs, cats, cattle, sheep, goats, and horses; and an inactivated tissue-culture vaccine has been made available for protecting people likely to be exposed to infection.

Rabies virus has also been grown in human cells, and this could offer a safe means of vaccine production for human use, though probably too expensive for large-scale application.

There are other possibilities in vaccine production. In 1957 Dr Van den Ende and colleagues reported that by centrifuging suspensions of infected mouse brains, the supernatant fluid could be used as an immunising agent.

Miss Joan Crick, MSc and Dr F. Brown reported (1969) that, working with killed Flury LEP virus, they had found it possible to protect mice with a vaccine made from particles smaller than those of the complete virus, and that such mice survived a challenge with live virus. Perhaps one day human beings could be protected in a similar manner.

VACCINES FOR USE IN ANIMALS

There is not the same problem with vaccines intended for use in animals as there is with those prepared for human use; the main difference being that in veterinary medicine the treatment of bitten or otherwise exposed *unvaccinated* animals is seldom or never undertaken. The whole emphasis is upon immunising animals against possible subsequent infection. The long course of injections, the serious side-effects are therefore avoided.

Japan is believed to have been the first country to have used dog vaccination on a large scale for the purpose of rabies control. A Semple-type vaccine, of rabbit brain origin, was developed in the early 1920s, and Japanese success with it aroused interest in the USA, where valuable research on methods of assessing the potency of this type of vaccine, and on establishing the duration of immunity in vaccinated dogs, was carried out.

In 1948 Dr H. Koprowski and Dr H. R. Cox developed a vaccine prepared from the Flury strain of virus (isolated from a girl victim of the disease in Georgia, USA). They adapted this virus to chick embryos after it had been passaged by Dr N. H. Johnson through 136 day-old chicks.

It was later demonstrated that the low-egg-passage (LEP) type of Flury vaccine—in which the virus had been passaged through 40-50 chick embryos—was more effective than the older types of inactivated-virus vaccines usually prepared from infected brains of sheep or goats. In fact, Flury LEP vaccine protected, in a trial, 100 per cent of dogs when challenged with rabies virus thirty-nine months after a single dose of the vaccine.

However, effective as it is in adult dogs, Flury LEP vaccine is not safe for use in puppies, or in species other than the dog.

Flury high-egg-passage (HEP) vaccine (involving 180 passages) is, on the other hand, safe for puppies, cats, and cattle.

Until the early 1960s, choice of vaccines for use in animals was limited to modified live Flury virus vaccine, or inactivated fixed virus vaccine of sheep or goat brain origin. Then came the introduction of inactivated cell culture vaccines, following Dr P. Fenje's work in Canada—to which reference has been made earlier in this chapter.

The ERA strain of virus, adapted by Dr Fenje to hamster kidney cells, was adapted by Dr Abelseth and colleagues to pig's kidney cells; and such a (live) vaccine has been used for the immunisation of dogs, cats, cattle, sheep, goats, and horses.

Other live tissue-culture vaccines have been prepared from the HEP-Flury strain of virus grown in dog's kidney cells; and from LEP-Flury strain virus grown in hamster's kidney cells.

Appendix B lists several of the anti-rabies vaccines currently in use for both human beings and domestic animals.

In Britain the Waterhouse Committee included in their (1971) Report the following extract from the WHO 5th Report:

> It is important to determine whether or not the living modified strain used in non-inactivated vaccine is excreted in the salivary glands of the species of animal for which the vaccine is designated. Since the pathogenicity of various modified strains of rabies virus for man is not known, excretion of such a strain in the saliva of the inoculated animal might create a public health hazard.

In view of this, and because of potential danger from live vaccine in pregnant animals or those under three months old, the committee did not recommend live vaccine for use in Britain.

Chapter Eight

The Human Patient

As mentioned in Chapter 2, man is an incidental rather than a maintenance host of the rabies virus; and the infection in man is a 'dead-end' one in that the human patient virtually never transmits infection to another person or animal.

An indication of the size of the rabies problem in human medicine is given by the fact that, in Europe—excluding East and West Germany—some 26,000 people undergo preventive treatment each year after exposure to rabies infection. In the USA the figure is about 30,000; in India 100,000.

It would be as erroneous to imagine that every person bitten by a rabid animal will himself become rabid if untreated as to imagine that every person who undergoes a course of treatment will necessarily escape the disease.

Dr A. D. Macrae stated (1970) that it has been estimated that 40-50 per cent of people bitten by a known rabid animal do not develop the disease even if untreated.

According to the Pasteur Institute, Teheran, wolf-bites may give rise to a mortality as high as 60 per cent; a reason being that bites from this animal so often involve severe lacerations inflicted on face or neck. Dr P. Lépine stated (1953) that although wolves were responsible for only 0·1 per cent of rabid animal bites, they caused 6·8 per cent of human deaths.

Wounds of the head, neck and shoulders are more dangerous, since the virus is deposited nearer to the brain, than those inflicted on the limbs.

In the USA, a Public Health Report states, over 51 per cent of those suffering from rabies, whose ages were known, were under fifteen years old. Various reasons can be advanced to account for this. Children tend to handle animals more than do adults; and sometimes children mistake rabid animals for tame ones and are bitten as a result. There is possibly a greater susceptibility to rabies at a younger age: a hypothesis reported by George Fleming as accepted in the last century. Then again, their shorter stature means that children are more likely to be bitten about the head than adults.

There are more cases of human rabies in the USA in spring, summer and autumn than in winter, probably because people engage in outdoor activities such as camping and picnicking which may bring them into contact with wildlife creatures suffering from the disease. The lighter clothing worn during the warmer months of the year will obviously offer less protection than heavy winter garb, and this factor may influence both the severity of bites and the quantity of virus infecting wounds.

Rabies is an exceedingly unpleasant disease, and one which has inspired dread for centuries. 'Its victims often die horribly, in great pain and distress,' commented the Waterhouse Committee (1971) in England; though they might have added that modern drugs can greatly alleviate that pain and distress.

With one possible recent exception in the USA, there has seldom or never been a case of recovery in the human patient which is regarded as fully authenticated today.

Pre-exposure inoculation

The nature of the disease, and the painful course of injections which comprise current treatment and which can lead sometimes to serious side-effects, are strong arguments in favour of people at risk, by reason of their occupation, receiving preventive inoculation. Such people include veterinarians, medical and veterinary research workers, laboratory technicians, and animal handlers such as the staff of quarantine kennels. Perhaps one should add to the list the keepers in zoological gardens; some of which have isolation premises authorised for quarantine purposes.

This protection involves two injections of vaccine at 4-6 week intervals, plus a booster dose after six months, and then annually; or three injections at weekly intervals plus a booster dose at three months, and then annually.

Dr A. D. Macrae commented: 'It is only after the booster that evidence of immunity in the shape of neutralising antibody is likely to appear, and even then it does not occur in 100 per cent of those inoculated.' He would regard this as a useful early step towards protection, but would insist on a full course in the event of exposure, at least until such times as more potent vaccines become available.

Pre-exposure preventive inoculation is not a new idea. Pasteur and his collaborators had already, in 1885, appreciated the need to protect those handling rabid animals and infected material. Two of Pasteur's assistants asked to be vaccinated, and duly received ten subcutaneous injections.

Pre-exposure vaccination was revived in the USA following work by Dr W. H. Dieterich and colleagues in 1961, and by Dr E. S. Tierkel and Dr R. K. Sikes, and by workers at the Pasteur Institute, Paris, in 1967.

Drs P. Lépine, P. Atanasiu, and A. Gamet stated (1971) that they had vaccinated 300 people without encountering any serious general reaction. Among those protected were seven who, without any doubt, were exposed to infection. Two injured their hands while opening skulls of rabid animals; and five pricked their fingers with hypodermic needles containing street virus.

Treatment after exposure

Dr P. R. Lépine, of the Pasteur Institute, has summarised the treatment of bitten persons under four headings as follows: (1) Cleaning of the wound. The use of soap and water or a detergent is usually recommended for this purpose; (2) the use of purified anti-rabies serum or, better still if available, human anti-rabies gamma-globulin. This is given by intra-muscular injection and also infiltrated around the wound(s); (3) after a lapse of twenty-four hours following the administration of anti-serum or gamma-globulin, the first dose of a vaccine of recognised efficacy and safety is given, to be followed by not less than thirteen further doses. Usually this course of fourteen or more injections are given on consecutive days; (4) booster dose(s) of vaccine in accordance with medical advice.

It is important to obtain treatment as soon as possible after the bite or scratches have been inflicted by a rabid animal, or after the latter's saliva has come in contact with eyes, lips, nose, sores or cuts on the skin (as discussed in Chapter 5). A doctor should be consulted even if the saliva has come into contact only with the unbroken skin.

The need for urgency in treatment was stressed by the British Medical Journal (1970), which cited a report from Vietnam of a soldier who was bitten on the finger and died of rabies 108 days later in spite of a full course of treatment begun within about thirty-six hours of his being bitten. 'His death was attributed to the thirty-six-hour delay in starting treatment.'

A fluorescent antibody test will normally show whether the biting animal is, in fact, rabid, and the test result can be available to the physician the same day that the specimen is received. Confirmation of the result is obtained later by mouse inoculation. (The fluorescent antibody test could be negative and the mouse test still positive, so that while a positive result with the former test confirms the need for treatment, a negative result is not necessarily an indication that treatment can be dispensed with.)

There is some danger of anaphylactic shock resulting from the use of antiserum obtained from horses (or sheep), and it has been recommended that a skin test for sensitivity in the patient be carried out before administration of antiserum.

Another unwelcome side-effect is serum sickness, which may appear from eight to twelve days after treatment begins. This condition, less severe than anaphylactic shock, may affect from 12 to 46 per cent of patients. WHO reported 2,367 cases of serum sickness among 21,870 patients who received antirabies serum during 1967.

Accordingly, the replacement of antiserum obtained from horses or sheep by a purified anti-rabies gamma-globulin of human origin—such as has been prepared at the USA Center for Communicable Disease Control—represents an important advance in the treatment of people exposed to rabies infection; making treatment less hazardous. At the time of writing, supplies are very limited, and increasing them will depend upon the willingness of people, who have been vaccinated against rabies but not exposed to a natural infection, to act as blood donors.

Effectiveness of treatment

How effective is present-day treatment in preventing the onset of rabies in human beings exposed to infection? This is a difficult question to answer with any degree of certainty, since controlled experiments with the rabies virus in human beings are not acceptable. In the absence of such experiments one can only quote the views of various authorities. Dr M. M. Kaplan has referred to the virtual elimination of deaths in eastern Mediterranean countries as a result of the combined use of anti-rabies serum and vaccine. Formerly, many people died from rabies in this region.

Professor Tierkel has commented that antiserum can help in head-bite cases in which, before its use, there was not sufficient time for the vaccine to exert a protective effect.

A very cautious note is sounded by a USA Public Health Report for 1967, which states that preventive treatment after exposure prevents some cases of the disease in man, 'particularly in persons for whom longer incubation periods would be expected.'

Dr A. D. Macrae, lately of the Virus Reference Laboratory, London, has commented that a combination of anti-rabies serum followed by a full course of vaccine, including booster doses, has been found effective after severe lacerating injuries. But he added: 'Even with this vigorous regimen, failures—with extended incubation periods up to 368 days after the bites—have been recorded.'

Antibody, stated Dr Macrae, is likely to be useful only when present in excess and in contact with extra-cellular virus at the site of infection during the very short period before infectious particles pass to the spinal cord and brain.

Once the virus is inside cells, antibody is believed to be ineffective. Moreover, during the usual course of treatment with vaccine, antibody is not generally detectable during the first ten days or fortnight. How then does this treatment prove effective? Professor C. Kaplan has suggested that the killed or attenuated virus particles in the vaccine may attach to and block the specific receptors on nerve cells involved with the uptake of virus.

According to this hypothesis, if enough receptor sites are

blocked between the entry wound and the central nervous system, the virus would not be able to progress centrally and the disease would not then appear.

Sometimes, however, the rabies virus may gain access to the central nervous system via the bloodstream; so that it would appear that the peripheral nerves do not constitute the sole route.

Vaccines

The Waterhouse Committee stated in their report that only some 80 per cent of those vaccinated have developed neutralising antibodies within one month of completion of their course of inoculations. 'Antibody tests should always be made and, where necessary, additional booster doses given until neutralising antibodies are detected.'

The report adds that experiments with cell culture vaccines have shown that a high level of antibodies may be produced in monkeys after only a single inoculation—a fact which encourages the hope that a similar result may be achieved in man within a few years.

Duck-embryo vaccine has been used extensively in the USA and elsewhere, and in the UK has likewise been preferred to vaccines of nervous-tissue origin, owing to the smaller risk of serious complications. Doubts have, however, been expressed from time to time as to the potency of duck-embryo vaccine; that is, its ability to stimulate production in the patient of virus-neutralising antibodies in adequate amounts. Dr A. D. Macrae commented (1971), 'Although I agree it is not particularly potent, duck-embryo vaccine is probably the best commercial vaccine presently available.'

Although duck-embryo vaccine is regarded as safer than vaccines made from nervous-tissue, Professor M. A. Selimov, Chief of the Laboratories for the Prevention of Rabies, Moscow, commented at the 1968 WHO Frankfurt conference that vaccine of duck origin could promote generalised reactions and might affect the nervous system, though less frequently than vaccine prepared from nervous tissue.

Dr R. K. Sikes considers that the factor which may bring about the complication of allergic encephalomyelitis is probably the myelin of the mammalian nervous tissue present in nerve-tissue vaccines of the Semple type.

The Pan American Zoonoses Centre, Buenos Aires, has reported that, as compared with adults, children very rarely develop allergic encephalomyelitis following vaccination with Semple nervous-tissue vaccine; and their susceptibility to allergic neuritis after inoculation with Fuenzalida vaccine (described in Chapter 7) is also lower than that of adults.

In 1967 WHO figures showed that there were 123 cases of paralysis out of 559,848 people who received vaccine treatment after exposure to rabies infection. This is fortunately a small percentage but that, of course, is no comfort to the people who suffered in this way. What is encouraging is the prospect of far safer vaccines becoming available within a very few years.

Rabies in man

The incubation period of rabies in man varies from six days to about two years. In a series of 137 cases in the USA, incubation periods ranged from 6 to 270 days, with an average of 37 days.

It was found that people who suffered multiple or exceptionally deep, lacerating bites, or face or head bites, usually had shorter incubation periods than those whose exposure to infection took a less severe form. For example, 53 of the 137 people whose injuries came into the former category had incubation periods of 6 to 156 days, with an average of 22 days. Among 18 people who had single bites below the neck, scratches, or licks on fresh wounds, incubation periods ranged from 20 to 270 days, with an average of 58 days.

The symptoms of rabies in man include fever, headache, nausea, a sense of apprehension, a burning sensation at the site of the bite, and muscular spasms when attempting to drink. These spasms may be extremely painful, and may later occur at the mere sight of water—a fact which led to the old name for the disease: hydrophobia.

In some cases there is extreme sensitivity to bright light. The patient may retain his mental faculties for much of the time, but there may be periods of mania during which he becomes destructive and tears bedclothes, for example. The voice may become hoarse, and he may emit strange sounds before the onset of the muscular spasms already referred to. There may be delirium, an extending paralysis, and convulsions before death. (In rabies arising from the bite of a vampire bat, the illness is paralytic in character, with little or no excitement, and no hydrophobia.)

The length of the illness in a series of 154 cases was found to vary between one and twenty days, with an average of four days.

In California in 1969 a boy, under three years old, died of rabies after an illness lasting 133 days—the longest ever recorded. He had been bitten on the head by a bobcat (lynx) which was killed and found positive for rabies. Treatment was begun on the day of the bite, but did not include antiserum; two doses of duck-embryo vaccine being given daily for seven days, with single doses on seven subsequent days, and booster doses on the twenty-first and thirty-first days.

Seventeen days after being bitten, symptoms appeared—fever and lethargy, followed a few days later by paralysis of both lower extremities. This paralysis extended upwards, but at no time was there difficulty in ingesting fluids or solid foods.

The patient remained alert until the twenty-fifth day, when stupor was followed by coma. Four days later, spontaneous breathing ceased and a respirator was brought into use.

In July 1970 there were two fatal cases of rabies in the USA, both resulting from skunk bites. In South Dakota a four-year-old boy was bitten, and immediately taken for medical treatment. Two bite wounds on the arm and multiple scratches around the child's face were found. The first daily dose of duck-embryo vaccine was given four hours after the bite. Nine hours later, 1,000 units of equine anti-rabies serum was injected intramuscularly, but none was infiltrated around the wounds. The boy became ill a little over four weeks after being bitten, and died about a week later.

The second case involved an eleven-year-old boy camping in Arizona. The skunk entered the boy's sleeping bag, and bit him first on his shoulder and then several times on his left hand. The animal remained in the sleeping bag until captured by the boy's father. Eight hours after the bites (which occurred at 1 am) the wounds were dressed, but vaccine treatment was not begun until about eighty hours had elapsed. Symptoms appeared in just over three weeks. Ten days later he died.

The US Department of Health commented: 'PHS Advisory Committee on Immunization Practices recommends for treatment of a severe, unprovoked bite by a wild animal 1,000 international units of equine anti-rabies serum per 40lbs of body weight, with half of the dose given intramuscularly and the remainder infiltrated at the site of the wound as soon after the bite as possible. In addition, 21 daily doses of DEV plus boosters on days 31 and 41 after the initiation of the series are recommended. These cases did not receive this optimal recommended therapy.'

Recovery from rabies

What is described as 'the first well documented recovery from rabies in world medical literature' formed a happier outcome for a six-year-old boy in Ohio. While he was in bed asleep, a bat (*Eptesicus fuscus*) which had apparently entered the room through an opening to the attic, bit him on the left thumb; from which the creature was pulled by the boy's father.

The bat was subsequently shown to be rabid by the fluorescent-antibody test on brain material, and also by mouse inoculation.

The bite wound was washed with soap and water. Anti-rabies serum was not given, and it was not until four days after the bite that the boy was started on a 14-day course of duck-embryo vaccine. Two days after the 14th dose, symptoms appeared—first, pain in the neck, and over the next several days lethargy, malaise, and loss of appetite. He was admitted to hospital with a temperature of 104°F. Over the next ten days this declined, but lethargy and neck stiffness were noticed. Walking and writing became difficult, the boy no longer spoke, behaved strangely and responded only to repeated requests. Weakness of his left arm, leg and face followed. 'The patient was in and out of coma for a week and then gradually began to improve', states the report. Nine days after being able to sit up in bed and feed himself, he was able to talk—in a high-pitched voice—and to walk unaided. Within three weeks he was able to run and speak in a normal voice. He was discharged from hospital on 27 January 1971 'with no neurological abnormality and has remained well'.

Intensive care was given, especially in assisting breathing and preventing a lack of oxygen, during his illness, and it is thought that these measures may have contributed to the arrest of the illness and eventual recovery.

Rabies virus was not isolated from the patient, but extremely high neutralising antibody titres against rabies—and their persistence—are regarded as strong evidence of infection; the titres being higher than the rabies vaccine would be expected to give rise to. Moreover, extensive tests were made for other viral and bacterial agents known to cause encephalitis, with negative results.

Conclusion

In summarising the position of the human patient today, it can be said that treatment after exposure prevents at least some cases of rabies; that serious side-effects do sometimes occur, especially following the use of vaccines made from nervous tissue; but that in a few years we should see revolutionary changes in post-exposure treatment, which will cease to be an ordeal to undergo and be both safer and more effective.

Table 8

The number of treated people bitten by various animals in thirteen countries, 1969:

Cameroon*	by dogs (1,453), rodents (35), cats (23), monkeys (17), others (5)
Congo, People's Republic of	„ dogs (515), monkeys (22), cats (13), rats (2), civet cat (1), guinea-pig (1), squirrel (1)
Costa Rica	„ dogs (1,558), rats (116), cats (63), squirrels (12), bats (7), monkeys (6), others (7)
France	„ dogs (478), cats (108), foxes (79), cattle (80), rats (12), monkeys (6), roe deer (5), martens/stone martens (8), badgers (2)

Guatemala	by dogs (1,278), rodents (29), cats (19), cattle (5), racoons (2), squirrels (2), coatimundi (2), pig (1), bat (1), horse (1)
India**	„ dogs (6,036), cats (27), cattle (26), buffalo (5), jackals (4), donkeys (2), rat (1)
Iran	„ Dogs (773), cats (82), wolves (35), jackals (4), others (42)
Italy	„ dogs (269), cats (58), rats (13), hamsters (14), rabbits (10), squirrels (6), monkeys (5), dormouse (1)
Mexico	„ dogs (42,142), cats (1,060), rats (550), bats (268), polecats (45), horses (32), pigs (18), squirrels (13)
Spain	„ dogs (1,437)
Sudan	„ dogs (1,260), camel (1), monkey (1)
Turkey†	„ dogs (7,561), cats (1,912), rodents (332), monkeys (66), bears (11), wolves (4), jackals (3), foxes (2), ruminants (37), solipeds (146), others 42)
Yugoslavia	„ dogs 1,827), cats (291), rodents (32), foxes (16), pigs (7), bears (5), horses (4)

*Notified via Pasteur Institute only.

**ditto. Figures from Kasauli Research Institute include additionally over 56,000 people bitten by dogs and 41 by foxes and wolves.

†Notified by Istanbul Institute only.

Appendix A

The Rabies Virus

Virology is a fast growing science, and it is barely possible to quote a text-book definition of viruses without grave risk of it being challenged by the time it reappears in print. Similarly there is a pitfall associated with the classification of viruses. In the 1960s the rabies virus was classified as a myxovirus. All one can say in 1972 is that it is currently classified as a RNA-containing virus and a member of the Rhabdovirus group. This name is taken from the Greek word for a rod, and the group includes—in addition to the rabies virus—at least thirty other bullet-shaped viruses with hosts as varied as the potato, rainbow trout, mosquito, horse, bat, and lettuce.

The rabies virus measures about 180mμ in length, with a diameter of about 75mμ (10mμ=0·00001mm). For purposes of comparison one may add that one of the smallest viruses, that causing foot-and-mouth disease, measures only 24mμ; while if one turns to bacteriology one finds that a staphylococcus is about 1,000mμ long.

Apart from its 'flat' end, which is actually concave or even hollow, the surface of the rabies virus is covered with projections. In the photograph of the model (see page 33) these have the appearance of spikes, but in reality the virus' projections each have a small knob at the end.

The particles, it seems, are not invariably bullet-shaped. Long rods and bell-shaped forms have also been described.

When the membranous covering or envelope of the virus is ruptured, a ribbon-like internal component is released. Part of this is composed of RNA (ribonucleic acid).

The virus particles can be photographed with the electron microscope but cannot be seen through the ordinary light microscope. However, what are technically known as virus-matrix complexes are formed when, for example, mouse brain is infected with 'street' virus; and these virus-matrix complexes, after appropriate staining, can readily be seen with the ordinary microscope. They have been shown by Drs Miyamoto and Matsumoto to be identical with Negri bodies, the finding of which in brain tissue has since 1903 constituted one means (and, until the introduction of the fluorescent antibody test, a very important one) of diagnosing rabies at *post-mortem* examination.

They also found that infection with 'fixed' virus gives rise to smaller virus-matrix complexes, and suggest that the 'fixed' virus damages nerve cells to such an extent that the development of typical Negri bodies does not occur.

The virus matures by budding at the cell surface or cytoplasmic membrane.

'Rabies-like' isolates

Recently some 'rabies-like' isolates have been made; for example, from bats in Nigeria and from voles in central Europe. These viruses apparently have longer incubation periods in experimental animals than most rabies strains, but do show some serological cross reactions with rabies virus. The exact inter-relationships have yet to be established.

More detailed information on the rabies virus will be found in the following:

Matsumoto, S. (1962) *Virology 17* 198

Miyamoto, & Matsumoto, S. (1967) *J.Exp.Med. 125* 447

'Advances in Virus Research' 1970, edited by Kenneth M. Smith, Max A. Lauffer & Frederick B. Bang. (Academic Press)

Appendix B

Some Officially Approved Vaccines

Some examples of officially approved Rabies Vaccines used in various countries—

Vaccines for use in human beings

Type	Tissue used	Virus	Inactivated by
DEV	duck embryo	fixed	betapropiolactone
Semple	rabbit/goat/sheep brain	fixed	phenol
Fuenzalida	suckling mouse brain	fixed	ultra-violet rays

Vaccines for use in domestic/farmyard animals

INACTIVATED

Type	Inactivator	Origin	For use in	Virus
Semple	phenol	sheep/goat brain	all domestic animals	fixed
Cell culture	various	hamster kidney		fixed
Cell culture	betapropiolactone	hamster kidney	cat, dog	fixed

LIVE

Type	Origin	Virus	Egg passage	For use in
LEP	Chicken embryo	Flury	40-60	dog (not puppies)
HEP	Chicken embryo	Flury	180 plus	cat, dog, and cattle
Kelev	Chicken embryo	Kelev	60-70	dog, cattle,
Cell culture	pig kidney cells	ERA		all domestic animals
	dog kidney cells	HEP-Flury		cat, dog, and cattle
	hamster kidney cells	LEP-Flury		dog
	chicken embryo cells	LEP-Flury		dog

Glossary

Anaphylactic shock	This may follow injection of a protein foreign to the body.
Antibody	A substance in the blood-serum or other body fluids formed to neutralise viruses, bacteria, etc.
Attenuation	The process of reducing the virulence of viruses, bacteria, etc.
Antiserum	Blood serum containing antibody to a specific virus, bacterium, or toxin.
Autonomic nerves	Those concerned with breathing, the beating of the heart, and other actions not under control of the will.
Carrier state	An animal recovered from a disease, or not showing symptoms, but capable of passing on the infection to another animal.
Central nervous system	The brain and spinal cord.

Challenge	To test the degree of immunity of an animal against a particular infection, eg by inoculating a dose of virulent virus into an animal already vaccinated against it, thereby determining the efficacy of the vaccine.
Conjunctiva	The mucous membrane lining the eyelid.
Cornea	The transparent window in the sclerotic coat of the eyeball.
Cupping	Bleeding by means of a cupping glass.
Encephalomyelitis	Inflammation of the nervous tissues of both the brain and spinal cord.
Endemic	Regular occurrence of a disease in a country or region.
Eosin	A red dye used for staining of cells/tissues.
Epithelial	Relating to the epithelium, the layers of cells covering the skin and lining the mouth, internal organs, etc.
Epizootic	A term applied to a disease which is affecting a large number of animals over a large area of land at the same time, and spreading rapidly.
Fixed virus	Virus which has been passaged through a number of, say, rabbits; becoming in

K

	the process more virulent for them but less so for other species, and giving rise to a reduced incubation period of rabies. Fixed virus apparently cannot multiply in salivary glands.
Fluorescein	A red, crystalline powder used in solution as a dye for diagnostic purposes. It fluoresces in the presence of ultra-violet light.
Gamma-globulin	A preparation of the protein fraction of the blood serum containing antibody.
Inclusion body	Round, oval, or irregular-shaped structures found in cells during the course of virus infections.
Incubation period	The time which elapses between infection and the appearance of symptoms of a particular disease.
Indirect transmission	Transmission of infection between two animals which have never been in physical contact.
Intracerebrally	Direct into the cerebrum, a part of the brain.
Myelin	The white, fat-like substance forming a sheath round myelinated nerve fibres.
Neutralising antibody	A defensive substance produced by the body against, for example, a virus, and rendering the latter incapable of attack.

Passage	(Pronounced as in French.) Passing a strain of organisms through a series of animals in order to decrease the virulence of that strain for another species —a technique of attenuation used in vaccine production.
Peripheral nerves	Those which lead to or from the brain and spinal cord.
Prophylaxis	Measures to ward off disease.
Serological	Relating to serum.
Serum sickness	An illness which may follow injection of a serum obtained from another species of animal. For example, an antiserum obtained from a horse may in some people give rise to fever, glandular enlargements, pain in joints, etc, some 8-12 days after the injection.
Street virus	The naturally occurring, as opposed to the fixed, rabies virus.
Titre	The extent to which an antibody-containing serum can be diluted before losing its power to react with a specific antigen, eg the rabies virus. 'High titres' means, in practical terms, that a patient's blood serum contains high levels of antibody.
Trachea	The windpipe.

Virion	A fully mature virus.
Virus	An infective agent, potentially disease-producing, which can multiply only in a living cell. (This, however, is not the full technical definition.)

SYNONYMS FOR RABIES

Canine Madness

Hydrophobia

Lyssa (Greek)

Rabbia (Italian, Spanish)

Rage (French)

Tollwut (German)

Acknowledgements

I should like to offer my thanks to Mr A. D. Irvin, MA, VetMB, MRCVS, of the East African Research Organisation, Kenya, for permission to abstract freely from his excellent paper on wildlife rabies in the *Veterinary Record,* and for the wealth of references to original source material; to Professor Franz Steck, University of Bern, for welcoming me to his laboratories, information, and for kindly reading with a critical eye Chapters 2, 3, 4, 5, and 7; to Dr A. D. Macrae, Consultant Virologist, City Hospital, Edinburgh, for allowing me to quote from recent papers of his and for reading Chapter 8; to Miss Joan Crick, MSc, and to Dr F. Brown, of the Animal Virus Research Institute, Pirbright, for kindly reading Chapter 7 and for other help; to Dr R. K. Sikes, Assistant Chief, Office of Veterinary Public Health Services, Atlanta, Georgia, for much information on the rabies situation in the USA and on rabies vaccines; to Professor C. Kaplan, University of Reading, for permission to quote from two recent papers of his; to Dr J. Muller, of the State Serum Laboratory, Copenhagen; to the World Health Organisation, Geneva, for use of their world surveys of rabies, scientific papers, and photographs; to Miss B. Horder, BA, Librarian of the Royal College of Veterinary Surgeons and staff; to the Pasteur Institute, Paris; to the British Veterinary Association for permission to quote from its publications; and to many others.

References

Chapter 1

Almeida, J. D. *et al* (1962) *Virology 18* 147

Country Life (1966) 930

Fleming, George (1872) *Rabies and Hydrophobia*

Hydrophobia—cases and cures selected from the Gentlemen's Magazine (1807)

Irvin, A. D. (1970) *Veterinary Record 87* 33

Kaplan, C. (1971) *Proc. roy. Soc. Med. 64* 228

Locke, J. & Dixon, W. T. (1965) *A Man of Sorrow*

Mead, Richard (1720) *A short discourse concerning pestilential contagion and the methods to be used to prevent it*

'Scrutator' (1852) *Letters on Hunting*

Snyman, P. S. (1937) *Journal S. Afr. vet. Med. Ass. 8* 126

Spackman, Thomas (1613) *A declaration of such grievous accidents as commonly follow the biting of mad dogs, together with the cure of*

Stratton, Julia (1960) *Vet. Rec. 72* 734

Tierkel, E. S. (1959) Advances in Veterinary Science

Youatt, William (1845) *The Dog*

Chapter 2

Anon (1960) *Bull. Off. int. Epizoot 60* 239

Anon (1968) *J. Amer. vet. Med. Assoc. 153* 871

Beauregard, M. (1969) *Can. J. Comp. Med. 33* 220

Bouffard, G. (1912) *Ann. Inst. Pasteur* 26 727

Boulger, L. R. (1966) *Lancet 1* 941

Cifuentes, C. (1967) *Bull Off. int. Epiz.* 67 467

Constantine, D. G. & Woodall, D. F. (1966) *Amer. J. vet. Res* 27 24

„ (1966) *Ibid. 27* 16

„ & Soloman, G. C. & Woodall, D. F. (1968) *Ibid 29* 181

Cooper, J. E. (1966) *Vet. Rec. 78* 435

Courtois, G. (1967) *Bull. Off. int Epizoot. 67* 457

D'Souza, B. A. *et al* (1968) *Ind. vet. J. 45* 633

Frye, F. L. & Cucuel, J. P. E. (1968) *J. Amer. vet. Med. Ass. 153* 189

Gottal, C. (1967) *Bull. Off. int. Epizoot. 67* 463

Held, J. R. Tierkel, E. S. & Steele, J. H. (1967) *Pub. Hlth. Rep. 82* 1009

Irvin, A. D. (1970) *Vet. Rec. 87* 333

McMillan, B. & Boulger, L. R. (1960) *Ann. trop. Med. Parasit. 54* 165

Martinez, C. R. (1963) *Bull. Off. int. Epizoot. 60* 131

Mohan, R. N. (1968) *Vet. Bull. 38* 587

Neitz, W. O. (1967) *J.S. Afr. vet. Med. Ass. 38* 129

Pawan, J. L. (1936) *Ann. trop. Med. Parasit. 30* 101

„ (1936) *Ibid. 30* 401

Schmidt, R. C. & Sikes, R. K. (1968) *Am. J. vet. Res. 29* 1,843

Sharp, J. C. M. (1967) *Brit. Med. J 3* 20
Sikes, R. K. (1962) *Am. J. vet. Res. 23* 1,041
„ (1971) Personal communication
Smith, P. C. *et al* (1967) *Nature 216* 384
Snyman, P. S. (1937) *J.S. Afr. vet. Med. Ass. 8* 126
„ (1940) *Onderstepoort Journal 15* 9
Steck, F. (1968) *Vet. Rec.* 83 Clin. Suppl. No. 15
„ (1971) Personal communication
Thiery, G. (1959) *Bull. epizoot. dis. Afr.* 7 265
Walker, V. C. R. (1969) *Can. vet. J. 10* 11
USA Annual Rabies Summary (1969)
WHO Monograph No 19
„ (1968) *Surveillance and control of Rabies*
„ (1970) *WHO Chronicle* 2 47

Chapter 3

Bedford, P. G. G. & Clarke, E. G. C. (1972) *Vet. Rec. 90* 53
Bouffard, G. (1912) *Ann. Inst. Pasteur 26* 727
Brown (1969) *Vet. Rec.*
Chalmers, A. W. & Scott, G. R. (1969) *Trop. Anim. Hlth. Prod. 1* 33
Gamet, A. & Toma, B. (1970) *Bull. Acad. Vet.* XLIII
Irvin, A. D. (1970) *Vet. Rec. 87* 33
Kaplan, C. (1970) *Science Journal* 6 32
Morgan-Jones, K. R. (1969) *Vet. Rec.*
Neitz, W. O. (1967) *J.S. Afr. vet. Med. Ass. 38* 129
Peace, C. K. & Hopes, R. (1969) *Vet. Rec. 87* 299

Serie, C. & Andral, L. (1963) *Ann. Inst. Pasteur 104* 123

Sikes, R. K. (1970) *Am. J. Pub. Hlth. 60*

Snyman, P. S. (1940) *Onderstepoort J. 15* 9

Steck, F. (1968) *Vet. Rec. 83* Clin. Suppl. No 15

Thiery, G. (1959) *Bull. epizoot. Dis. Afr. 7* 265

Tierkel, E. S. (1959) *Adv. vet. Sci. 5* 183

USA Annual Rabies Summary 1969

WHO World Surveys of Rabies

Wright, J. Mrs (1970) *Vet. Rec.*

Report of the Committee of Inquiry on Rabies (HMSO, London, 1970)

Chapter 4

Jordan, W. J. & Hosseinion, M. (1965) *Vet. Rec. 77 789*

Mohan, R. N. (1968) *Vet. Bulletin 38* 67

Morehouse, L. G. *et al* (1968). *J. Amer. vet. Med. Ass. 153 57*

Report of the Committee of Inquiry on Rabies (HMSO, London, 1971)

Schnurrenberger, P. R. *et al* (1970) *J. Amer. vet. Med. Ass. 156* 1455

Sikes, R. K. (1970) *Amer. J. Pub. Hlth. 60*

Snyman, P. S. (1940) *Onderstepoort J. 15* 9

Steck, F. (1968) *Vet. Rec. 83* 10

Tierkel, E. S. (1959) *Adv. vet. Sci. 5* 183

Walker, V. C. R. (1969) *Can. vet. J. 10* 11

WHO Expert Committee on Rabies (1966)

" World Surveys of Rabies 1967, 1969

Chapter 5

Annual Rabies Summary (1969) (US public health report)

Fleming, George (1872) *Rabies and Hydrophobia*

Constantine, D. G. (1966) *Am. j. vet. Res. 27* 16
„ Solomon, G. C. & Woodall, D. F. (1968) *Am. j. vet. Res. 29* 181

Crick, J. & Brown, F. (1971) Personal communication

Hole, N. H. (1969) *Nature 222* 244

Irvin, A. D. (1970) *Vet. Rec. 87* 333

Kaplan, M. M. (1970) *Proc. roy. soc. Med. 64* 225
„ WHO Monograph No 19

Macrae, A. D. (1969) *Lancet* 1,415

Parker, R. L. & Wilsnack, R. E. (1966) *Am. j. vet. Res. 27* 33

Report of the Committee of Inquiry on Rabies (HMSO, London, 1971)

Sikes, R. K. (1962) *Am. j vet. Res. 23* 1,041
„ (1970) *Am. j Public Health 60*

Steck, F. (1968) *Vet. Rec. 83* Clin. Suppl. No 15
„ (1971) Personal communication

Sully, Henry (1807) *Hydrophobia*

Tierkel, E. S. (1959) *Adv. vet. Sci. 5* 183

WHO Chronicle June 1971

Chapter 6

Aruo, S. K. (1971) *Veterinary Record* 79

A History of the Overseas Veterinary Services, *Part 1, 1961

Ballantyne, E. E. & O'Donoghue, J. G. (1954) *J. Am. vet. Med. Ass. 125* 316

Hooton, A. E. (1970) Personal communication

Report of the Committee of Inquiry on Rabies (HMSO, 1970)

Sikes, R. K. (1970) *Am. J. Pub. Hlth. 60*

„ (1971) Personal communication

Muller, J. (1971) Personal communication

USA Public Health Report—*Annual Rabies Summary 1969*

WHO Chronicle (1970) *24* 7

„ World Surveys of Rabies, 1967, 1969

„ Frankfurt-on-Main conference report, 1968

Yasmuth, Chamroon *et al* (1970) *Lancet* 1313

(*a BVA publication, edited Geoffrey P. West)

Chapter 7

Anon (1971) *Vet. Rec.* Supplement *89* 194

Atanasiu, P. Gamet, A. & Virat, B. (1968) *Q.S. Vétérinaire 8* 94

Crick, J. & Brown, F. (1969) *Nature 222* 92

„ „ (1970) *Lancet* 1,106

Comptes Rendues des Séances de l'Académie des Sciences, Paris, 1885

Held, J. R. Tierkel, E. S. & Steele, J. H. (1967) *USA Public Health Report 82* 11

Kaplan, C. (1970) *Science J. 6* 32

„ (1971) *Proc. roy. Soc. Med. 64* 228

Macrae, A. D. (1971) Personal communication

Parish, H. J. *A History of Immunization*

Sikes, R. K. (1969) *Arch. Environmental Hlth. 19*

WHO report of Frankfurt-on-Main conference (1968)

„ *Chronicle* (1971) *25* 250

USA Public Health Service Report (1969)

References

Report of the Committee of Inquiry on Rabies (HMSO, London, 1971)

Chapter 8

Anon (1970) *Brit. Med. J.* 2 742

Crick, J. & Brown, F. (1970) *Lancet* 1,106

Kaplan, C. (1970) *Science Journal* 6 32

Lépine, P. (1953) WHO Monograph No 19
„ *et al* (1971) *J. de Therapeutique 3*

Macrae, A. D. (1969) *Lancet* 1,415
„ (1970) *Health Trends* 2 58
„ (1971) Personal communication

Report of the Committee of Inquiry on Rabies (HMSO, London, 1971)

Sikes, R. K. (1971) Personal communication

Tierkel, E. S. (1959) *Adv. vet. Sci.* 5 813

USA Annual Rabies Summary 1969, 1970

WHO Chronicle (1966) *20* 449
„ Report on Frankfurt Conference
„ World Surveys of Rabies 1967, 1968

Index

Index

Index